Second Edition

KT-529-475

Motivating People to Be Physically Active

Physical Activity Intervention Series

Bess H. Marcus, PhD

Program in Public Health
Brown University

LeighAnn H. Forsyth, PhD

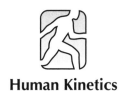

Human Kinetics

Library of Congress Cataloging-in-Publication Data

Marcus, Bess, 1961-
    Motivating people to be physically active / Bess H. Marcus, LeighAnn H. Forsyth. -- 2nd ed.
        p. ; cm. -- (Physical activity intervention series)
    Includes bibliographical references and index.
    ISBN-13: 978-0-7360-7247-2 (soft cover)
    ISBN-10: 0-7360-7247-0 (soft cover)
    1. Exercise therapy. 2. Exercise--Psychological aspects. 3. Motivation (Psychology) 4. Health
behavior. 5. Physical education and training. I. Forsyth, LeighAnn, 1967- II. Title. III. Series.
    [DNLM: 1. Physical Fitness. 2. Exercise. 3. Health Behavior. 4. Motivation. 5. Program Devel-
opment. QT 255 M322m 2009]
    RM725.M373 2009
    615.8'2--dc22

                                                            2008023195
ISBN-10: 0-7360-7247-0
ISBN-13: 978-0-7360-7247-2

Copyright © 2009, 2003 by Bess H. Marcus and LeighAnn H. Forsyth

All rights reserved. Except for use in a review, the reproduction or utilization of this work in any
form or by any electronic, mechanical, or other means, now known or hereafter invented, including
xerography, photocopying, and recording, and in any information storage and retrieval system, is
forbidden without the written permission of the publisher.

Notice: Permission to reproduce the following material is granted to instructors and agencies who
have purchased *Motivating People to Be Physically Active, Second Edition:* pp. 66, 69, 73, 76, 77,
84-87, 91, 168-176. The reproduction of other parts of this book is expressly forbidden by the above
copyright notice. Persons or agencies who have not purchased *Motivating People to Be Physically
Active, Second Edition,* may not reproduce any material.

The Web addresses cited in this text were current as of August 2008, unless otherwise noted.

Acquisitions Editor: Michael S. Bahrke, PhD; **Developmental Editor:** Kathleen Bernard; **Assistant
Editors:** Jillian Evans, Scott Hawkins, and Kyle G. Fritz; **Copyeditor:** Patsy Fortney; **Proofreader:**
Julie Marx Goodreau; **Indexer:** Sharon Duffy; **Permission Manager:** Dalene Reeder; **Graphic
Designer:** Bob Reuther; **Graphic Artist:** Dawn Sills; **Cover Designer:** Keith Blomberg; **Photogra-
pher (cover):** Neil Bernstein; **Photographer (interior):** © Human Kinetics, unless otherwise noted.
Photos on pages 7 and 79 © Photodisc, photo on page 49 © 2001 Brand X Pictures, photo on page 61
© Eyewire; **Photo Asset Manager:** Laura Fitch; **Photo Office Assistant:** Jason Allen; **Art Manager:**
Kelly Hendren; **Associate Art Manager:** Alan L. Wilborn; **Illustrators:** Alan L. Wilborn and Dick
Flood; **Printer:** United Graphics

Printed in the United States of America   10 9 8 7

The paper in this book is certified under a sustainable forestry program.

Human Kinetics
Web site: www.HumanKinetics.com

United States: Human Kinetics
P.O. Box 5076
Champaign, IL 61825-5076
800-747-4457
e-mail: humank@hkusa.com

Canada: Human Kinetics
475 Devonshire Road, Unit 100
Windsor, ON N8Y 2L5
800-465-7301 (in Canada only)
e-mail: info@hkcanada.com

Europe: Human Kinetics
107 Bradford Road
Stanningley
Leeds LS28 6AT, United Kingdom
+44 (0)113 255 5665
e-mail: hk@hkeurope.com

Australia: Human Kinetics
57A Price Avenue
Lower Mitcham, South Australia 5062
08 8372 0999
e-mail: info@hkaustralia.com

New Zealand: Human Kinetics
P.O. Box 80
Torrens Park, South Australia 5062
0800 222 062
e-mail: info@hknewzealand.com

Second Edition

Motivating People to Be Physically Active

Withdrawn

ACCESSION No. T060974

CLASS No. 796.01

To my late mother, Betty, whom I miss so much, for her support and love and for always inspiring me to do my best; to Amber, our newest addition, welcome and thanks for all of your smiles, hugs, and kisses; to my husband, Dan, for his constant love, support, and positive energy; to my awesome big kids, Brittany and Josh, who make each day an adventure and who keep me on my toes!

—BHM

To my husband, Paul, for always sticking by me and providing me with love and support whenever I need it; to my mom, Wilma, and my late father, Jim, who have always supported me in whatever I choose to do; and to my kids, Olivia, Evan, and Owen, who never fail to bring me perspective and make life so much more fun!

—LHF

CONTENTS

PART I   Theoretical Background and Tools for Measuring Motivational Readiness   1

CHAPTER 1   Describing Physical Activity Interventions. 3

CHAPTER 2   The Stages of Motivational Readiness for Change Model 11

CHAPTER 3   Integrating Other Psychological Theories and Models. 21

viii ■ CONTENTS

CHAPTER 4 **Putting Theories to Work by Looking at Mediators of Change** **35**

Consider Mediators of Physical Activity Behavior Change 36
Factors That Enhance Physical Activity 38
Unlock the "Black Box" 46
Conclusion 47

CHAPTER 5 **Using the Stages Model for Successful Physical Activity Interventions.** **49**

Imagine Action: A Community-Based Program 50
Jump Start to Health: A Workplace-Based Study 52
Jump Start: A Community-Based Study 54
Project Active: A Community-Based Study 55
Project STRIDE: A Community-Based Study 56
Step Into Motion: A Community-Based Study 56
Conclusion 57

PART II Applications 59

CHAPTER 6 **Assessing Physical Activity Patterns and Physical Fitness** **61**

Discovering Patterns of Physical Activity Behavior 62
Determining Intensity Level 63
Tracking Physical Activity Behavior 65
Assessing Fitness 73
Assessing Physical Activity and Fitness in Group Settings 77
Conclusion 78

CHAPTER 7 **Using the Stages Model in Individual Counseling** . . **79**

Physical Readiness 80
Physical Activity History 82
Psychological Readiness 82
Confidence 89
Set Short- and Long-Term Goals 90
Measure Success 91
Conclusion 108

CHAPTER 8 **Using the Stages Model in Group Counseling Programs** **109**

Leading a Stage-Based Group 110
Learning From a Sample Stage-Based Curriculum 115
Assessing Your Effectiveness as a Leader 118
Conclusion 128

BISHOP BURTON COLLEGE

SERIES PREFACE

The purpose of the Physical Activity Intervention Series is to publish texts, written by the leading researchers in the field, that provide specific and evidence-based methods and techniques for physical activity interventions. These books include practical suggestions, examples, forms, questionnaires, and intervention techniques that can be applied in field settings.

Many health professionals who currently provide exercise advice and offer exercise programs use the traditional and structured frequency, intensity, and time (FIT) approach to exercise prescription. Although the exercise prescription is valid, going to a fitness facility and participating in such programs are not attractive to many people. Alternative programs based on the new consensus recommendations and using behavioral intervention methods and techniques are needed.

The books in the Physical Activity Intervention Series provide information, methods, techniques, and support to the many health professionals—clinical exercise physiologists, nutritionists, physicians, fitness center exercise leaders, public health workers, and health promotion experts—who are looking for alternative ways to promote physical activity that do not require a rigid application of the FIT approach. It is to meet this need that Human Kinetics developed this Physical Activity Intervention Series.

The series has a broad scope. It includes books focused on after-school programs for children and youth, ways to implement physical activity interventions in the public health setting, and ways to evaluate physical activity interventions. The series also includes books that focus on the implementation of interventions based on theories and on interventions for other special populations such as older adults and those with chronic disease. Each book is valuable and useful in its own right, but the series will provide an integrated collection of materials that can be used to plan, develop, implement, and evaluate physical activity interventions in a wide variety of settings for diverse populations.

o writing this book was to translate these ca

PREFACE

Our purpose in writing this book was to translate theories and concepts from behavioral science research into a handbook useful for health professionals who are involved in planning, developing, implementing, or evaluating physical activity programs. Our hope is that *Motivating People to Be Physically Active* will be useful for you if you are a personal trainer, an employee at a health club or community center, or a staff member at a community or federal agency, or if any aspect of your job involves helping people increase their motivation for behavior change, especially behavior change related to physical activity. We have filled this book with practical tools, case studies, ideas, and methods that you can readily use no matter how much you know or do not know about the fields of psychology and behavior change.

You may choose to read this book in its entirety, or you may choose to read just the chapters that are most relevant for your work. However, we hope that you will become familiar with the concept of motivational readiness so that you can use this book as a reference for ideas and strategies for putting those ideas into practice. The skills, tools, and strategies presented here can be used in individual, group, workplace, or community settings.

Although the aim of *Motivating People to Be Physically Active* is to provide you with knowledge, skills, and resources for working with healthy adults, you can apply the information presented here to whatever population you work with, including populations with chronic physical or psychological conditions.

In the first part of the book, we focus on the foundations of research on physical activity interventions, tools for measuring motivational readiness for behavior change, and mediators of behavior change. In chapter 1 we differentiate physical activity programs from other programs that pertain to exercise and fitness training. In chapter 2 we introduce the stages of motivational readiness for change model, the theoretical model that serves as the foundation of much of this book. In this chapter we also discuss how to measure motivational readiness for change. In chapter 3 we discuss other influential psychological theories and models and their applications to physical activity interventions. In chapter 4 we describe mediators of change for physical activity behavior, which is what needs to change before a person can change his or her physical activity behavior. We also describe how to measure these mediators of change. In chapter 5 we review successful physical activity intervention studies that have used the stages of motivational readiness model.

In part II we describe the assessment of patterns of physical activity and physical fitness, and we also look at applications of the stages of motivational readiness model to various settings. In chapter 6 we describe how to measure your clients' physical activity patterns and physical fitness. In chapters 7 through 10 we discuss how to apply the stages of motivational readiness model to individual, group, work site, and community settings. We also discuss how you can apply these concepts to specific populations. Within these chapters we also provide exercises and worksheets that you can use in your physical activity programs and case studies that we hope will give you some ideas of how you might use the information presented.

We wish you much success in your work helping people to be physically active. We applaud you for focusing your time and energy on this critically important area of health promotion and disease prevention.

ACKNOWLEDGMENTS

Before we mention the various people who have assisted us with this project, we first want to acknowledge that the writing of this book, while challenging, was fulfilling and sometimes downright fun because of the close professional and personal relationship we have with each other. Working on this book while we each held down full-time jobs and took care of our kids was only possible because we supported and laughed with each other during the process.

Several people have assisted us with various aspects of this project. We thank Shira Gray for helping us with formatting the chapters and tracking down important articles for us. We thank Zoe Bruno for helping us stay on track during the editing process. We also thank Joe Ciccolo, PhD, and Dori Pekmezi, PhD, for their helpful comments on various sections of the book.

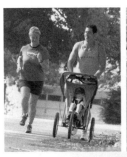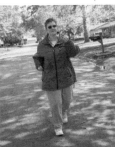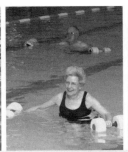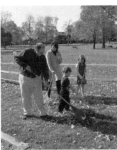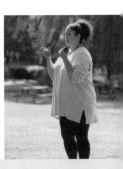

Theoretical Background and Tools for Measuring Motivational Readiness

The focus of the first part of this book is on the foundations of research on physical activity behavior, physical activity interventions, tools for measuring motivational readiness for behavior change, and mediators of behavior change. This part also describes the public health recommendations for participation in a physically active lifestyle and the types of activities that can be performed at a moderate intensity. We explain the health benefits of participating in physical activity as well. Finally, we describe the differences between physical fitness, exercise, and physical activity and explain the importance of theory-based interventions aimed at the promotion of a physically active lifestyle.

PART one

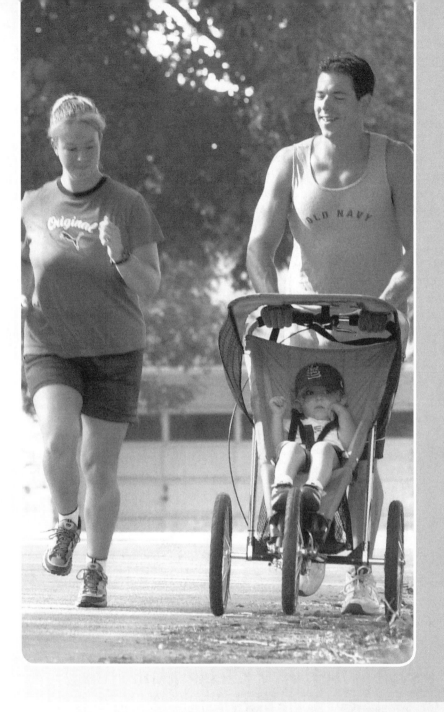

CHAPTER 1

Describing Physical Activity Interventions

Sedentary living is a leading cause of poor quality of life, disability, and death in the United States and many other countries. Numerous well-conducted research studies on this topic have been completed over the past 50 years, providing convincing evidence of the important physiological and psychological changes that occur during and following exercise training programs. Over the past 25 years numerous public health organizations, including the American Heart Association (AHA), the American College of Sports Medicine (ACSM), the Centers for Disease Control and Prevention (CDC), the National Institutes of Health (NIH), and the Surgeon General's office, have released statements regarding the health benefits of an active lifestyle and the health consequences of a sedentary lifestyle (Fletcher et al., 1992; Haskell et al., 2007; NIH, 1996; Pate et al., 1995; U.S. Department of Health and Human Services [USDHHS], 1996, 2000). These statements are based on examinations of population-based studies that consistently found that physical activity or physical fitness reduces the risk of cardiovascular disease in a dose-response manner. That is, those who have the greatest fitness or participate in the greatest amount of physical activity have the lowest risk. These studies also found that those who perform moderate amounts of activity or who are moderately fit also have a large reduction in their risk for cardiovascular disease relative to sedentary people. Following is a list of the health benefits acquired through an active lifestyle.

Benefits of physical activity

Reduced risk of heart disease, high blood pressure, and diabetes

Reduced risk of colon cancer

Reduced risk of breast cancer

Healthy and strong bones

Less chance of catching colds and flu

Better weight management

Increased energy

Better sleep

Less anxiety and depression

Enhanced self-esteem

Physical Activity Recommendations

Data from various studies have allowed researchers to develop guidelines for the amount of exercise needed to create and maintain these health benefits. Findings from these studies led the ACSM to develop the exercise prescription with which many of you are already quite familiar (see table 1.1). It is currently recommended that people accumulate 30 minutes or more of at least moderate-intensity (60 to 74% of their maximum heart rate) physical activity on at least 5 (preferably all) days of the week, or at least 20 minutes of at least vigorous-intensity (75 to 85% of maximum heart rate) physical activity on 3 or more days per week (ACSM, 2000).

TABLE 1.1   **Exercise Recommendations for Improved Overall Health**

Intensity	Duration	Frequency	Examples
Moderate (60-74% of maximum heart rate)	30 minutes or more in one long bout or several 10-minute bouts	5 or more days of the week	• Brisk walk for 30 minutes • 10 minutes of walking, 10 minutes of raking, 10 minutes of playing tag with the kids
Vigorous (75-85% of maximum heart rate)	20 minutes or more	3 or more days of the week	• Jogging for 20 minutes • Spinning class

Reprinted, by permission, from W.L. Haskell et al., 2007, "Physical activity and public health, updated recommendation for adults from the American College of Sports Medicine and the American Heart Association," *Medicine and Science in Sports and Exercise* 39: 1423-1434.

In addition to these population-based studies, several experimental studies led exercise scientists to examine the effect of intensity level as well as the minimum length of each bout of activity. A study by DeBusk, Stenestrand, Sheehan, and Haskell (1990) revealed that several short bouts (e.g., three 10-minute bouts) of moderate-intensity to vigorous-intensity activity in a day produced similar improvements in health-related outcomes to one longer bout (e.g., one 30-minute bout). Another study by Ebisu (1985) demonstrated that three shorter sessions of exercise resulted in similar improvements in fitness and greater improvements in HDL cholesterol than one or two longer sessions. Thus, both vigorous- and moderate-intensity activity have important health implications, as do both continuous and accumulated bouts of activity.

These findings have resulted in health organizations making recommendations for health-promoting physical activity: Adults should accumulate at least 30 minutes of at least moderate-intensity physical activity on at least 5 days of the week (Haskell et al., 2007; Pate et al., 1995). Moderate-intensity activities are those that require exerting some effort but not pushing oneself as hard as more vigorous-intensity activities such as running. We often tell clients that a good example of moderate-intensity activity is brisk walking; that is, walking with a purpose, as though you were late for a meeting, trying to catch a bus, or hurrying to get out of the cold. For health benefits moderate-intensity activities should be performed for at least 10 minutes at a time. More examples of moderate-intensity physical activities are listed on page 6. You may have also heard about the weight control recommendations listed in table 1.2. These are from the U.S. Department of Health and Human Services, which recommends 30 minutes of physical activity per day to prevent chronic disease and at least 60 minutes per day to manage weight (USDHHS & USDA, 2005). In addition to the recommendations for aerobic activity listed earlier, it is recommended that adults and especially older adults also do strength building (resistance training) activities 2 to 3 days per week, as well as stretching exercises to increase flexibility on a daily basis (Nelson et al., 2007; USDHHS, 1996).

TABLE 1.2   **Physical Activity Recommendations for Weight Control**

Desired goal	Minimum duration	Minimum intensity
Maintenance of current weight	60 minutes/day	Moderate
Prevention of weight regain	60-90 minutes/day	Moderate

USDHHS. *Dietary guidelines for Americans,* 2000. Washington, D.C.; USDHHS, Report of the Dietary Guidelines Advisory Committee.

Examples of moderate-intensity physical activities

Bicycling

Brisk walking (15-20 minutes per mile)

Dancing

Gardening and yard work

Golf (without a cart)

Hiking

Playing actively with children

Playing volleyball

Raking leaves

Vacuuming a carpet

Washing and waxing a car

Definitions of Physical Activity, Exercise, and Physical Fitness

Probably because they are used to the former recommendations that focused only on vigorous exercise with the goal of fitness change, many health professionals and laypeople alike use the terms *physical fitness, physical activity,* and *exercise* interchangeably, although their actual meanings are not the same. Perhaps you also substitute these terms for one another. You will notice that throughout this book we emphasize *physical activity* as opposed to exercise or physical fitness, in keeping with the new physical activity recommendations. We believe that the distinctions among these terms are critical, so let us clarify what each means before proceeding:

- *Physical fitness* is an outcome that can be attained through exercising at the frequency, intensity, and length of time prescribed by the ACSM (2000).
- The term *physical activity* refers to any bodily movement that results in the burning of calories (Caspersen, 1989).
- *Exercise* is actually a subcategory of physical activity; it is physical activity that is planned, structured, and repetitive.

The focus of this book is developing programs that help people to increase *daily physical activity* rather than, or in addition to, planned exercise. Activities such as taking the stairs more often at work, raking leaves in the yard, and shooting baskets with the kids should be included as successful outcomes of programs such as those described in this book. A sedentary person who never liked vigorous exercise may be more accepting of a physical activity program that encourages strategies such as these.

Following are some strategies for meeting the CDC/ACSM public health recommendations:

- Taking one 30-minute walk each day for at least 5 days of the week
- Taking one 30-minute walk on each weekend day and three 10-minute walks a day on at least 3 weekdays
- Doing three 10-minute bouts of activity on at least 5 days of the week (a sample day might include 10 minutes of digging in the garden, a 10-minute brisk walk to the post office, and 10 minutes of playing tag with the kids)
- Doing 30 minutes of heavy housework on one day, 30 minutes of heavy yard work on another day, and 3 days of accumulating at least 30 minutes of brisk walking in blocks of time that are at least 10 minutes in duration

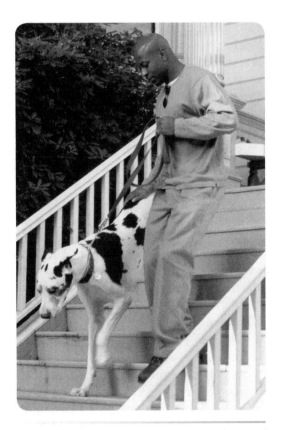

To help meet the CDC/ACSM public health recommendations, engage more frequently in some outdoor hobbies that you enjoy, such as walking and playing with the dog.

You, as a health professional, are on the front line, working with people to change their behavior. Thus, these more recent recommendations are really written for you so that you can truly have a wide array of options for working with individuals, groups, or communities. We believe that most people will be much more responsive to your program offerings or individual coaching if you share with them this newer public health approach and the notion that they do not need to engage in intense, "no pain, no gain" workouts to reap all the benefits of a physically active lifestyle. In fact, by giving people the choice to accumulate their activity over the course of a day or to do it all at once, to do a moderate-intensity activity such as brisk walking or a more vigorous activity such as running, and to participate in physical activity at a gym, community center, or their own neighborhood, you give them enough tools to succeed at adopting and maintaining a physically active lifestyle, perhaps for the first time in their lives.

Physical Activity Interventions

Despite the numerous benefits of physical activity and the recent attention to specific guidelines, only 32% of U.S. adults (based on *Healthy People 2010* guidelines) engage in regular leisure-time physical activity (Barnes & Schoenborn, 2003). Given the many benefits of physical activity and the low prevalence rates, it is imperative that interventions be designed that effectively promote the adoption and maintenance of active lifestyles for the approximately 50 million Americans who are sedentary and at high risk for chronic disease or functional limitations (Marcus et al., 2006; USDHHS, 1996, 2000).

Moreover, because of the many social disparities (e.g., in age, income level, and education level) in the segments of the population that are sedentary, interventions that do not rely solely on costly face-to-face contact with a health or fitness professional are critical. Many people cannot afford to join a health club or community center. People in lower income brackets are also less likely to see a primary care doctor on a regular basis than are those in higher income brackets. Thus, these people are not well served by current facilities and organizations. This has led behavioral scientists and public health researchers to develop effective interventions that can be delivered through other channels, such as the Internet, telephone, pamphlets distributed within the community, and programs offered at the workplace (Marcus, Nigg, Riebe, & Forsyth, 2000; Marcus et al., 2007a, 2007b).

Exercise training studies are typically conducted at gyms and supervised by health professionals. In exercise training studies, the goal is to determine the physiological effects of various amounts of exercise. Psychological theory is often not the framework on which these studies are based. In contrast, the goal for physical activity interventions is to help people change their behavior and replace sedentary pursuits with active ones. For example, helping people to choose to meet friends for walks or bike rides rather than lunch or coffee might be one of the goals of a physical activity intervention. The goal of physical activity interventions is to help people reorient their lives to include physical activity.

Physical activity promoters are increasingly recognizing that to keep people active, they need to help them develop physical activity habits that fit their lifestyles. For example, for a person who works at the office from 8 a.m. until 8 p.m., having home exercise equipment may be the only way to structure the environment so that regular physical activity is an option. Of course, simply having exercise equipment in the environment does not provide the motivation for the person to actually use it. For that, the person may need to learn to pair leisure activities he likes and perceives as important, such as watching the evening news, reading the newspaper, or listening to music, with the use of the home exercise equipment. In this way, hopping onto the treadmill at 8:30 p.m. can be something to look forward to all day rather than one more thing to get through on a busy day.

Those who design physical activity interventions have also learned the importance of helping clients discover activities that they enjoy. Teaching people that activities they consider fun, such as dancing and gardening, can count toward the daily goal of accumulating 30 minutes of moderate-intensity activity is a great way to get people who otherwise might not take up regular exercise to at least consider doing so. Interventionists and program planners have also become aware of the need to design programs that are flexible enough to accommodate changes in their clients' life circumstances and routines. For example, jump rope classes at health clubs and workplace wellness centers provide the skill and the proper equipment for people to be physically active in any location. Since a jump rope can easily be packed into a briefcase or a small bag, clients can carry it wherever they are throughout the day until it is time for a jump rope class.

Theoretical Models

Studies have shown that in randomized trials people often do better long-term if they are in home-based programs (King, Haskell, Taylor, Kraemer, & DeBusk, 1991). Giving people the choice of gym-based or home-based exercise programs has advantages. Home-based programs offer the opportunity for continuous or intermittent bouts of practical activities such as yard work, housework, and gardening. As a result of the difference between home-based and gym-based programs, theoretical models that attempt to explain physical activity as a behavior and the factors that influence it have been central to physical activity intervention studies. For example, the stages of change approach, which examines people's motivation for changing their physical activity habits, the barriers that get in their way, the benefits they hope to glean from an active lifestyle, and the specific strategies and techniques for becoming more active, may help them achieve their goals. These parameters can be best addressed by applying psychological theories to the promotion of physically active lifestyles.

Motivational Readiness for Behavior Change

The stages of motivational readiness for change model (Prochaska & DiClemente, 1983) provides a framework for examining people's motivation for changing their physical activity habits, the barriers to change, the benefits of change, and specific strategies and techniques for promoting change. It is one of the four theoretical models highlighted in the recent U.S. surgeon general's report on physical activity and health (USDHHS, 1996). This model has great utility for those who work with individuals, groups, and communities because it highlights the need to assess both physical and psychological issues when designing programs. It also helps in the selection of strategies for behavior change that may be most useful for people with different levels of motivation to change. This theoretical framework is central to much of this book because it can help you understand how to motivate adults to be physically active.

Conclusion

In this chapter we have described the public health recommendations for participation in a physically active lifestyle. We have also reviewed examples of moderate-intensity physical activities and the health benefits of participating in such activities. We have explained the differences between physical fitness, exercise, and physical activity and have discussed the importance of theory-based interventions aimed at the promotion of a physically active lifestyle.

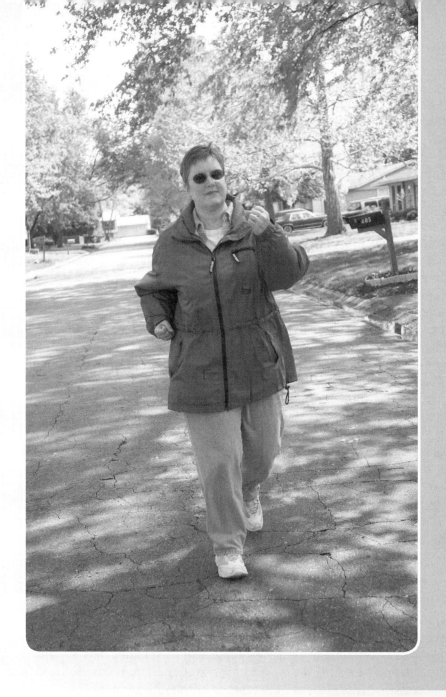

CHAPTER 2

The Stages of Motivational Readiness for Change Model

BISHOP BURTON COLLEGE

As you may know, approximately 25% of the American population is sedentary. In addition, 60% of Americans report not participating in recommended amounts of physical activity (USDHHS, 1996). In the programs you manage, you may encounter people who participate in some activity, such as a Thursday night bowling or softball league or tennis with a friend on Saturdays, but do not participate in physical activity on a frequent enough basis to reap health benefits. Because so many people are either inactive or infrequently active, effective programs to help them start and stick with an active lifestyle are critical.

Many of the techniques used to promote physical activity originated from psychological theories of motivation and behavior change. The stages of motivational readiness for change model, also known as the transtheoretical model or the stages of change model, evolved from the work of Dr. James Prochaska and Dr. Carlo DiClemente. Initially, they studied how people quit smoking on their own, without professional help (Prochaska & DiClemente, 1983). They were interested in learning how people change when they are not receiving help, thinking that this would provide valuable information to professionals who help others to change their health habits. Through their in-depth study of people who changed their smoking habits on their own, Drs. Prochaska and DiClemente learned that people moved through specific stages as they struggled to reduce the number of cigarettes they smoked or to quit smoking altogether. The model was initially labeled the transtheoretical model (Prochaska, 1979) because it was developed from many psychological theories, such as social cognitive theory (Bandura, 1977) and learning theory (Skinner, 1953).

Motivational Readiness and the Stages of Change

The key concept in the model that Prochaska and DiClemente developed is that of *stages of change,* and thus many people refer to the model as the stages of change model. We call it the stages of motivational readiness for change model to emphasize that this model focuses on both motivation for change and actual behavior change. It acknowledges that when attempting to make long-lasting behavior changes, people vary in their levels of motivation to change, from no intention to change to actually making behavior changes.

This model posits that there are five stages of readiness for change. For physical activity, the stages are defined this way:

▪ Those in the *inactive and not thinking about becoming more active* stage (stage 1) include people who do no physical activity and do not intend to start in the next 6 months. This stage is hereafter referred to as *not thinking about change.*

▪ The *inactive and thinking about becoming more active* stage (stage 2) applies to people who do not participate in physical activity but intend to start in the next 6 months. This stage is hereafter referred to as *thinking about change.*

▪ Those in the *doing some physical activity* stage (stage 3) participate in some physical activity but not at levels meeting the American College of Sports Medicine/American Heart Association (Haskell et al., 2007) guidelines of accumulating at least 30 minutes of at least moderate-intensity physical activity on 5 or more days of the week or at least 20 minutes of continuous vigorous exercise on at least 3 days per week, and they may or may not intend to become more physically active.

▪ People in the *doing enough physical activity* stage (stage 4) participate in recommended amounts of physical activity but have done so for less than 6 months and may or may not maintain this level of physical activity, as in they may or may not intend to or they may or may not be able to.

▪ Those in the *making physical activity a habit* stage (stage 5) have participated in recommended amounts of physical activity for 6 months or longer (Marcus & Simkin, 1993).

Movement through the stages is thought to be cyclical, rather than linear, because many people do not succeed in their efforts at starting and sticking with lifestyle changes (figure 2.1); in other words, people move back and forth among these stages (Prochaska, DiClemente, & Norcross, 1992). For example, if a person is in the thinking about change stage (stage 2) and moves straight into the doing enough physical activity stage (stage 4), accumulating at least 30 minutes of at least moderate-intensity activity at least 5 days a week, this may not result in long-lasting change. That is, if he skips over the stage of doing some physical activity (stage 3), he may not be adequately prepared for the rigors of daily activity, neither for the physical demand of that amount of activity nor for the time demand on his schedule. If he develops some foot or knee pain or decides that the 2 1/2 hours per week he is devoting to walking takes too much time away from work, he may say, "To heck with this physical activity. It just doesn't fit into my life, so I am not going to do it." The risk is that not only will he slide back to an earlier stage, but in fact he may slide right back to the not thinking about change stage rather than the thinking about change stage.

This model is also cyclical because changing a habit often takes many cycles before success is attained. That is, a person may need to make numerous attempts at behavior change before she is able to reach the making physical activity a habit stage (stage 5). You are probably quite familiar with the concept of one step forward and two steps back—this is often true for behavior change and may be quite frustrating for your clients.

Although the title of the fifth stage, making physical activity a habit, suggests that once a person reaches this level, she will maintain her physical activity

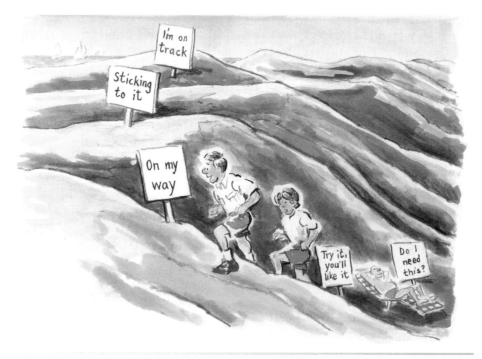

FIGURE 2.1 Movement through the stages is often cyclical rather than linear; people will often ebb through the stages.

Reprinted, by permission, from S.N. Blair et al., 2001, *Active living every day* (Champaign, IL: Human Kinetics), 8.

for the long term, there is a strong likelihood that she will slide back to earlier stages for periods of time. This sliding back could be due to competing demands on her time, her health, or a myriad of other reasons. Fortunately, research has shown that once a person reaches this stage, she is more likely to slide back to doing some physical activity (stage 3) or at worst to thinking about change (stage 2) and not all the way back to not thinking about change (stage 1) (Marcus, Selby, Niaura, & Rossi, 1992).

It is not known whether a person needs to remain in the making physical activity a habit stage (stage 5) for some critical period of time to reduce the risk of backsliding. In other words, it is not known whether there is a *termination* stage—that is, when participating in physical activity on a regular basis is simply a permanent way of life, but it seems unlikely. Even if a person truly enjoys the activity in which he participates and has participated in it on a regular basis for many years, he still needs to remain vigilant to ensure that he continues. It never ceases to be an issue in his life. This is important for program planners and those working with clients to keep in mind as they help people to make short- and long-term goals for physical activity. The stages of change are summarized in table 2.1.

TABLE 2.1   **Stages of Motivational Readiness for Change**

Stage number	Description
Stage 1	Inactive and not thinking about becoming more active
Stage 2	Inactive and thinking about becoming more active
Stage 3	Doing some physical activity
Stage 4	Doing enough physical activity*
Stage 5	Making physical activity a habit

*Accumulating at least 30 minutes of moderate-intensity physical activity at least 5 days per week

Match Treatment Strategies to Stages of Change

Most intervention programs are designed for people in the doing some physical activity stage (stage 3) or the doing enough physical activity stage (stage 4)—that is, people who are already engaged in physical activity. However, more than half the population is not in either of these stages. Therefore, those of us interested in helping people to lead more active lives need to think about other types of programs to offer those in stage 1 and stage 2. They are the ones who most need to change, yet few opportunities for change are offered to them, and they are not motivated enough to seek out opportunities on their own.

We studied a sample of participants in a workplace health promotion project (Marcus, Rossi, Selby, Niaura, & Abrams, 1992) and classified 24% as in stage 1, 33% as in stage 2, 10% as in stage 3, 11% as in stage 4, and 22% as in stage 5. Other samples in the United States and Australia have shown similar percentages. Our studies and those of our colleagues in the United States, Australia, and Europe have demonstrated that when there is a mismatch between participants' stages of motivational readiness for change and the intervention strategy used, they are more likely to drop out of the program; even if they stay in, they are less likely to reach their goals. For example, if a person still in stage 2 is given information appropriate for those in stage 4, such as specific tips on exercise programs, she may disregard the materials, intending to refer to them later, when or if she feels ready to start. This increases the chances that she will forget about the information she has received or decide that the program is not right for her because the material was not relevant to her level of motivation at that time. Matching treatment strategies to people's stages of motivational readiness for change improves the likelihood that they will attend a program regularly, increases their chances of meeting their short- and long-term goals, and decreases the likelihood that they will stop participating in the program or stop reading the materials provided.

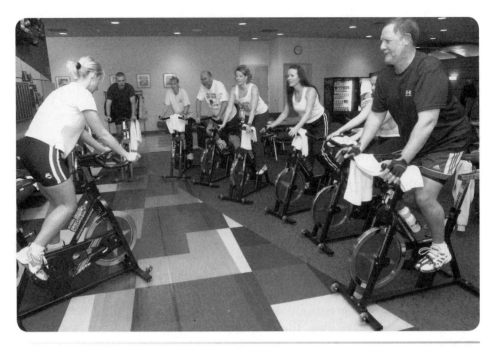

Traditional intervention programs often target those already motivated to become more physically active. Other types of programs may be needed for individuals in the earlier stages of change.

Processes of Behavior Change

The stages of motivational readiness for change model also addresses the processes of behavior change (Prochaska, Velicer, DiClemente, & Fava, 1988). These processes of change are the strategies and techniques that people use to modify their behavior. The original work investigating the processes of change, like that investigating the stages of change, was conducted on smokers and has since been extended to physical activity.

The stages of change explain *when* people change, and the processes of change describe *how* people change. Determining which specific processes of change to focus on with a given client depends on that client's stage of motivational readiness for change. Using a questionnaire we developed about processes of change for physical activity, we discovered that for physical activity, all of the processes are important at all of the stages of change (Marcus, Rossi, et al.,1992). Nonetheless, it is not feasible to emphasize all processes at each contact with a person, and thus key processes are usually selected based on the person's stage (Marcus et al., 1998).

Processes of behavior change are divided into two categories: cognitive (involving thinking, attitudes, awareness) and behavioral (involving actions).

The cognitive processes of change regarding physical activity are as follows:

- Increasing knowledge
- Being aware of risks
- Caring about consequences to others
- Comprehending benefits
- Increasing healthy opportunities

The behavioral processes of change regarding physical activity are as follows:

- Substituting alternatives
- Enlisting social support
- Rewarding yourself
- Committing yourself
- Reminding yourself

Questionnaire 4.1 for assessing these 10 processes of change (how much the client is using the process/strategy) can be found in appendix A. When people are in stage 2, they typically use mostly *cognitive* processes and some *behavioral* processes. People in stage 4 typically use mostly *behavioral* processes and some *cognitive* processes. These strategies and techniques for helping people to change their behavior were derived from a variety of psychological theories and models and are often used in counseling (Prochaska, 1979). Table 2.2 lists ways you can help clients to engage in the processes of change.

Programs based on the stages of motivational readiness for change model match treatment to the person's stage of readiness for change. For example, a stage-matched physical activity promotion intervention for people in the early stages of change (stage 1 or stage 2) might focus on increasing the use of the cognitive processes. Thus, the program might increase awareness of the benefits of physical activity and encourage thinking about becoming active. Materials designed for people in the later stages (stages 3, 4, and 5) can focus more on the behavioral processes. Such materials might encourage people to begin exercising and suggest strategies for maintaining an active lifestyle, such as rewarding oneself for reaching an activity goal or putting reminders to be active around the home and the workplace.

Working with clients on increasing their self-confidence regarding their ability to become and stay physically active is helpful (Bandura, 1977, 1986, 1997). It is also usually important to help clients understand more about the benefits of becoming physically active. Finally, because behavior change is not an easy process, practitioners can also work with clients on understanding and overcoming their personal barriers to behavior change (Janis & Mann,

TABLE 2.2   **Processes of Change**

Cognitive strategies	
Increasing knowledge	Encourage your client to read and think about physical activity.
Being aware of risks	Provide your client with the message that being inactive is very unhealthy.
Caring about consequences to others	Encourage your client to recognize how his inactivity affects his family, friends, and coworkers.
Comprehending benefits	Help your client to understand the personal benefits of being physically active.
Increasing healthy opportunities	Help your client to increase her awareness of opportunities to be physically active.
Behavioral strategies	
Substituting alternatives	Encourage your client to participate in physical activity when she is tired, stressed, or unlikely to want to be physically active.
Enlisting social support	Encourage your client to find a family member, friend, or coworker who is willing and able to provide support for being active.
Rewarding yourself	Encourage your client to praise himself and reward himself for being physically active.
Committing yourself	Encourage your client to make promises, plans, and commitments to be active.
Reminding yourself	Teach your client how to set up reminders to be active, such as keeping comfortable shoes in the car and at the office, ready to be used at any time.

1977). Often, components that address self-confidence, benefits, and barriers are used in combination with the stages and processes of change in individual, group, workplace, and community programs. Chapters 3 and 4 provide more information about self-confidence and the benefits of and barriers to physical activity. Information on measuring a client's stage of change is presented in the next section; information on measuring processes of change, self-confidence, barriers (cons), and benefits (pros) is also provided in chapter 4.

Determining a Client's Stage of Change

In this section we describe how to measure the stages of motivational readiness for change. The flowchart in figure 2.2 is a helpful visual aid for explaining the concept of stages of motivational readiness to your clients. Studies that have looked at the stages of change questionnaire (questionnaire 2.1 in appendix A) have found that people tend to get similar scores over a 2-week period (Marcus, Selby, et al., 1992). This gives us increased confidence that

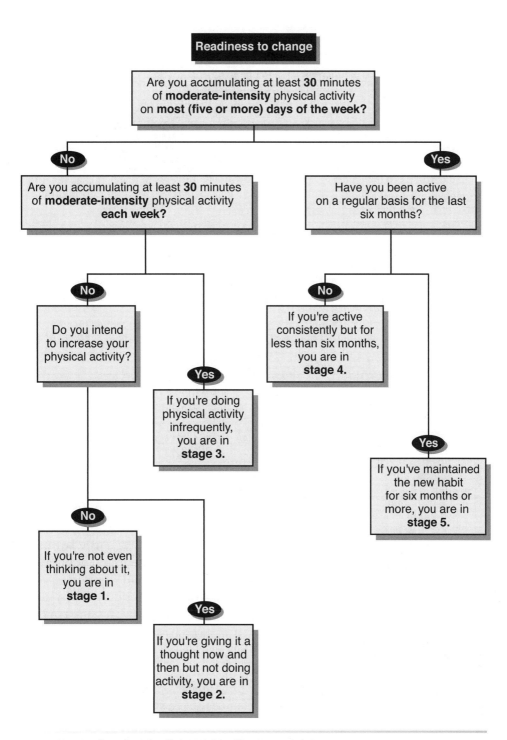

FIGURE 2.2 Flowchart for determining the stage of change.

Reprinted, by permission, from S.N. Blair et al., 2001, *Active living every day* (Champaign, IL: Human Kinetics), 9.

this questionnaire is measuring people's intentions and actual behavior in general, not just at the time they are filling out the questionnaire. We also have found that the questionnaire is related to measures of actual physical activity (Marcus & Simkin, 1993). This is important because it means that there is a direct relationship between a person's stage of motivational readiness for change and the number of minutes he is physically active each week. There is also a relationship between moving forward one or more stages and increases in physical fitness (Dunn et al., 1997). You can simply copy the questionnaire in appendix A for use with your clients.

Scoring the Stages of Change Questionnaire

Clients in stages 1 and 2 should have responded to questions 3 and 4 with zeros to ensure consistency in responses. In other words, clients who are inactive and either thinking about or not thinking about becoming active should answer no to questions 3 and 4, because it is impossible to not be physically active and to be physically active at the same time. Occasionally, clients answer yes to both, which indicates that they have not read the questions carefully or that they do not understand them. In this case, you should clarify the meaning of these questions for your client.

The scoring algorithm determines clients' particular stages at the time they complete the questionnaire only. However, this questionnaire has been shown to be stable over a 2-week period. When a client is found to be in stage 3 (doing some activity), 4 (doing enough activity), or 5 (making activity a habit), the second question (about whether she intends to increase her activity in the next 6 months) does not play a role in determining which stage she is in at the time she completes the questionnaire. This question is used to distinguish between clients in stage 1 (not thinking about becoming active) and stage 2 (thinking about becoming active). However, your client's intention to increase physical activity in the next 6 months can be highly relevant for intervention planning, and thus you may want to make a note of it. For example, if your client is in stage 3 (doing some activity) but answers that he is not planning to increase his activity over the next 6 months, you will probably want to ask him why he has sought your help. Perhaps he misunderstood the question. Or perhaps he came to see you only because his wife or his boss strongly encouraged him to do so, and he really has no intention of changing his behavior.

Conclusion

In this chapter we have described the concepts of motivational readiness and stages of change. We have discussed that this is a cyclical model and that programs work best when they are matched to a person's level of readiness to engage in behavior change. Additionally, the processes of change, or strategies and techniques for behavior change, have been described, and the concepts of self-efficacy and decision-making for behavior change have been introduced.

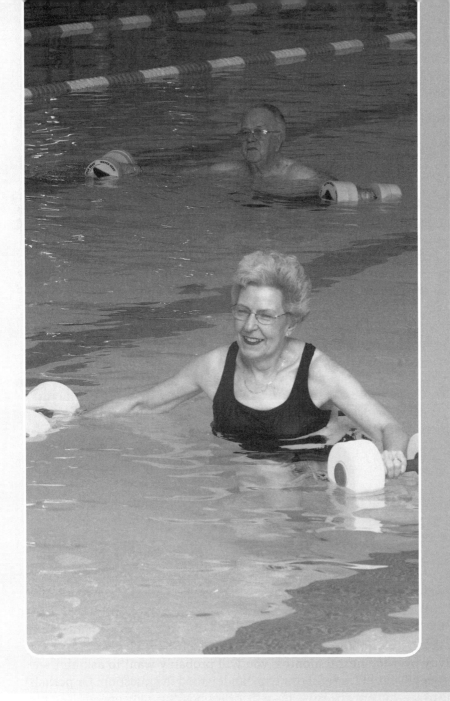

CHAPTER 3

Integrating Other Psychological Theories and Models

Physical activity includes many types of behavior, such as walking, playing volleyball with the kids, and raking the leaves in the yard. It also includes more traditional types of exercise, such as jogging and aerobics. Several factors seem to influence whether a person is physically active—self-confidence, the belief that she will gain something from activity, support from family and friends, and whether she enjoys active pursuits. Some health promoters have turned to psychological theories and models to better understand the many factors involved in starting to live an active lifestyle and maintaining physical activity behaviors. Theories from behavioral science also have been useful in developing, implementing, and evaluating health promotion efforts.

This chapter describes some psychological theories and models that can be useful when developing strategies for helping clients to become more physically active. We mention several of the most promising theories because no one model seems to fully explain physical activity and the ways we can most effectively help people to change this behavior. Some theories appear to be more appropriate for looking at physical activity at the individual level, whereas others are more applicable at the community level. A more comprehensive review of these theories and models can be found in chapter 6 of the 1996 U.S. surgeon general's report *Physical Activity and Health* (USDHHS, 1996).

Learning Theory

Behavior modification and learning theories (Skinner, 1953) have been widely applied to physical activity behavior change. According to learning theory, a person is more likely to be physically active when the right circumstances are in place and pleasurable consequences occur as a result of physical activity (figure 3.1). For example, a client is more likely to be physically active when a place to exercise is readily available, he has time set aside, and he has already experienced a sense of accomplishment after squeezing in 30 minutes of activity on a previous day. In turn, if this client finds activity rewarding, he will be more likely create the circumstances that will allow him to be active in the future.

Learning theory also acknowledges that when developing a new, complex behavior, such as physical activity, it is crucial to start with small steps and then progress slowly toward the desired result. This is called *shaping*. Often, newly physically active people start off by setting goals that are too difficult, such as walking every day for 45 minutes. Likewise, program developers often set up programs that are too frequent, long, or intense for those newly physically active, such as three 60-minute kickboxing classes per week. As a result, the new exerciser becomes frustrated or injured and thus drops out before the physical activity habit is established. However, by setting smaller, achievable goals (e.g., starting off with a 10-minute walk once a week, then gradually building to a 30-minute walk several times a week), the new exerciser can develop a sense of accomplishment and learn strategies for overcoming barriers that may have led to failure in the past.

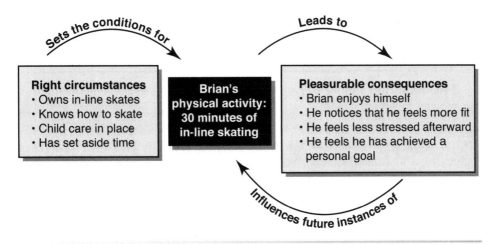

FIGURE 3.1   Learning theory.

By starting off with small goals (scheduling time, taking a walk even when tired, asking a family member to look after the kids for half an hour), your client can take steps that are necessary for regular physical activity. As she becomes skilled at each of these small steps, the goal is then gradually increased (e.g., adding 5 minutes of daily activity each week). A reward can be planned for each goal that is achieved.

It is critical that your clients understand the importance of starting off slowly. If they believe that starting slowly is a lesser approach to becoming more active and fit, they may disregard your program, which will then undermine their relationship with you and increase the likelihood that they will set themselves up for failure. For years people have been hearing "no pain, no gain," "go for the burn," and other messages that intense exercise in an all-or-none format is needed to gain benefits. We now know from the scientific literature that these extremes are not necessary for health. However, if your clients do not understand that your approach is consistent with the new recommendations and beneficial to their health, they may disregard your suggestions.

Learning theory also informs us that acquiring a new behavior typically requires frequent rewards and many pleasant consequences, at least in the beginning. This is particularly relevant to physical activity, which is often perceived as immediately punishing (e.g., time-consuming, painful, tiring), while many of its rewards (e.g., becoming healthier, feeling more energetic) do not occur for quite a while. Therefore, some programs have offered immediate rewards such as social praise or cash for participation until natural reinforcers such as stress relief and muscle tone are achieved. In fact, programs using reward strategies such as attendance lotteries, behavioral contracts, and tangible rewards (e.g., gift certificates for exercise clothes) have been found to increase regular exercise participation by as much as 75% in the short-term (King et al., 1992). For example, a program might allow participants to earn points for every half hour of activity, which they can cash in for exercise clothes or gift certificates.

However, programs based on extrinsic rewards do not seem to help people stay active over the long term (Glanz & Rimer, 1995). When a program that uses prizes to encourage participation or attendance ends, its participants tend to go back to their sedentary lifestyles. Therefore, it is important to also incorporate strategies that enhance natural rewards from exercise (e.g., encouraging participants to set up their own support networks or helping them find activities they enjoy and can see themselves doing for a while) so participants will be more likely to keep exercising after your formal involvement is over.

Although it is important for people to eventually experience intrinsic rewards (e.g., a feeling of accomplishment, enjoying the new look of one's body, or increased vigor), this can take quite some time, especially for clients who do not tend to use intrinsic rewards in other aspects of their lives. Reminders for physical activity can increase the likelihood that a person will become physically active. Drs. Brownell, Stunkard, and Albaum (1980) found that simply posting a sign near the stairs and elevator with a cartoon of a healthy heart climbing the stairs encouraged people to use the stairs rather than the elevator.

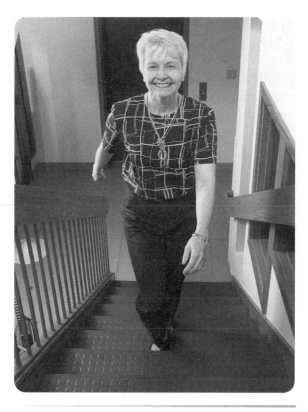

Taking the elevator is an unhealthy habit; taking the stairs is a healthy habit.

Decision-Making Theory

Decision-making theory attempts to explain how people decide whether to engage in a particular behavior based on their comparison of the perceived benefits versus the perceived costs of the behavior (Janis & Mann, 1977). In other words, we are more likely to be active if we believe that the benefits of being active (e.g., improved health, stress relief) outweigh the costs (e.g., time taken away from other activities, getting hot and sweaty) (figure 3.2). A person's weighing of the possible gains against the difficulties or losses experienced as a result of behavior change is often referred to as *decisional balance.*

People in the later stages of motivational readiness for change perceive more benefits of being physically active (more energy, less stress), whereas

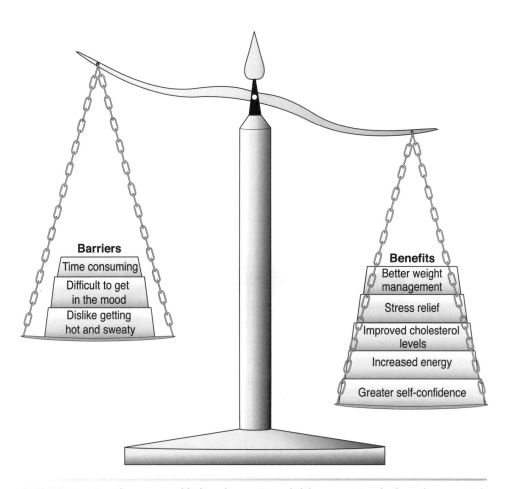

FIGURE 3.2 People are more likely to be motivated if they perceive the benefits outweigh the barriers.

people in the earlier stages perceive more disadvantages (uncomfortable, too time-consuming) than advantages (Marcus, Rakowski, & Rossi, 1992). One way you might use this theory in a program is to have your client write down what they think they will both gain and lose from participating in physical activity both in the short and long term. You can then use this list to begin discussing anticipated barriers and ways to increase perceived benefits (Marcus, Rakowski, & Rossi, 1992; Wankel, 1984). In appendix A, we provide a simple measurement tool (questionnaire 4.4) you can use with clients to assess their decisional balance toward physical activity.

Behavioral Choice Theory

Behavioral choice theory is based on decision-making theory but also incorporates research in the areas of learning, planning, and economics (Epstein, 1998). This theory attempts to explain how people decide among the behavioral options available to them and how they then use their time among various activities, both sedentary and active. According to this theory, people have a choice between being sedentary and being physically active, and this choice is influenced by many factors, such as the availability of physical activities versus sedentary activities, perceived benefits versus barriers, reinforcement (i.e., rewards, both tangible and perceived), and degree of effort (figure 3.3). For example, reducing the accessibility of sedentary behaviors (e.g., parking spaces that are close to the building) and increasing the cost of being sedentary (e.g., a staircase close to the building's entrance but the elevator down the hall so that it actually takes more effort to take the elevator than to take the stairs) are both methods for reducing sedentary behaviors.

Whether a client performs a behavior and whether he enjoys it depend partly on all the options available. For example, when your client comes home from a stressful day at work, he can plop down on the couch to watch TV, he can sit and talk to a friend on the phone, or he can go out for a brisk walk. If you and he can come up with an option that is both enjoyable and readily available, he may be able to choose an active pursuit rather than a sedentary one without having to throw the TV out or put a lock on the phone! For example, you might encourage your client to arrange to walk with a friend right after work as a way to relieve stress. You might encourage him to make his favorite sedentary activities dependent on doing some physical activity. For instance, if he enjoys reading each night, you might encourage him to not do this sedentary behavior unless he has done 30 minutes of physical activity that day.

Laboratory studies have shown that sedentary, obese children will spend time pedaling a stationary bike if they can also take part in their favorite sedentary behaviors such as playing video games or watching movies (Saelens & Epstein, 1998). However, for this strategy to work, the sedentary behavior must be one the person enjoys or engages in every day (Saelens & Epstein, 1999).

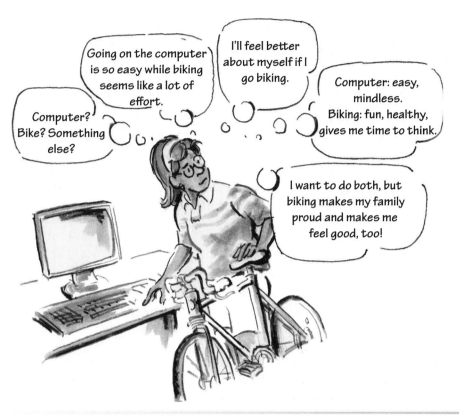

FIGURE 3.3 Behavioral choice theory.

Another important component of the behavioral choice theory is that for people to experience rewarding consequences as a result of physical activity, they need to believe that they are freely choosing to be active and are not being active only to please someone else. If people perceive that they are being forced to initiate an activity program rather than choosing on their own to become more active, they may not be motivated to change their lifestyles to more physically active ones. Discussing how your client can personally benefit from physical activity or allowing her to set her own goals for physical activity rather than giving her the goal you think is best can help her recognize that the choice of becoming active is hers.

Finally, choosing an active over a sedentary behavior depends in part on the time delay between making the choice and reaping the benefits from that choice. For physical activity, many of the benefits (e.g., less risk of developing heart disease) are delayed, whereas the benefits of being sedentary (e.g., having fun watching a movie on television) are immediate. Therefore, it is important to encourage your client to look for immediate, but often overlooked, rewards of being active (e.g., feeling energized, the pleasure gained from doing something good for oneself, being a good role model to friends and family) and to keep in mind the long-term effects of sedentary behaviors that are often forgotten at the moment of choice.

Social Cognitive Theory

Social cognitive theory (Bandura, 1986, 1997, 2001) has been applied most successfully to changing physical activity behavior. This theory proposes that behavior change is affected by interactions among the environment, personal factors, and attributes of the behavior itself, a concept which has been called *reciprocal determinism* (figure 3.4) (Bandura, 1986). In other words, each of these three forces may affect or be affected by the other two. Furthermore, making physical activity a regular behavior can result from direct reinforcement. For example, you might praise a client who has stayed with her program for 3 months. A person may also adopt habitual physical activity behaviors as a result of observing the consequences that others experience. For instance, Mary may decide to dust off her stationary bike after a friend has described how biking has helped her to feel less stressed and thereby to deal better with her kids, an issue that is also relevant for Mary.

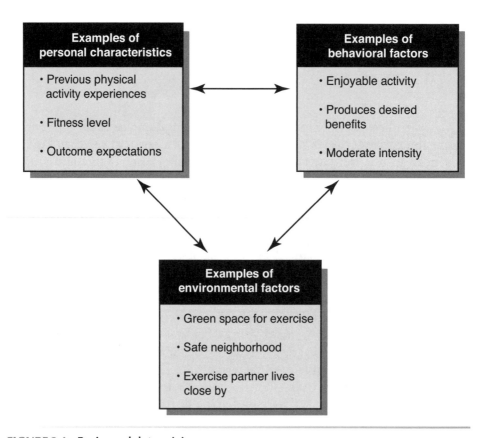

FIGURE 3.4 Reciprocal determinism.

A central concept in social cognitive theory is *self-efficacy,* or confidence in one's ability to successfully perform a particular behavior. People's perceptions that they can perform successfully increase the likelihood that they will engage in that behavior. Self-efficacy is behavior specific; for example, a person may be confident that he can cut down on his fat intake but not believe that he will be able to stay physically active. To be even more specific, he may feel confident that he can maintain a walking program but not feel confident that he could get himself to a gym four times a week for a fitness class. Self-efficacy has been shown to be related to physical activity behavior (Lewis, Marcus, Pate, & Dunn, 2002; Sallis et al., 1989); therefore, it is important to evaluate and, if necessary, improve a client's self-efficacy for the type of activity you are targeting. Measuring self-efficacy is discussed in chapter 4; the question-naire for self-efficacy (questionnaire 4.2) can be adapted for a specific type of physical activity (e.g., walking). Strategies for enhancing self-efficacy are included throughout part II.

According to social cognitive theory, a person must also believe that positive outcomes *(outcome expectations)* will follow if she is physically active and that these positive outcomes (e.g., weight maintenance, lower cholesterol) outweigh any negative outcomes she might also experience (physical discomfort during activity) (Bandura, 1997). The person must value these positive outcomes, whether they be short term (e.g., feeling more energetic following physical activity) or long term (e.g., warding off heart disease or diabetes).

Ecological Model

The ecological model seeks to explain behavior and behavior change in rela-tion to sociocultural and environmental variables. The basis of the ecological approach is that some environments restrict physical activities by promot-ing (and even demanding, in some cases) sedentary behaviors and limiting possible active pursuits (Badland & Schofield, 2005; Sallis, Bauman, & Pratt, 1998). For example, many workplaces are designed in such a way as to limit opportunities for physical activity. Often the elevator is in a central location, whereas staircases are in the far corners of the building, and many workplaces do not contain exercise facilities or walking space nearby. Although we still have much to learn regarding how people's physical environments affect their physical activity, many believe that environments can be designed to foster activity by including more green spaces, bike paths, and staircases that are safe, attractive, and easily accessible (Badland & Schofield, 2005; Humpel, Owen, & Leslie, 2002). This model states that it is important to develop physi-cal environments and policies that support activity, in addition to helping individuals develop personal skills, because there are multiple levels of influ-ence on physical activity (McLeroy, Bibeau, Steckler, & Glanz, 1988). Table 3.1 illustrates the levels of influence.

To change physical activity behavior, the program must be implemented on multiple levels. Programs that influence multiple levels and multiple settings

TABLE 3.1   **Components of the Ecological Model**

Components	Examples
Personal factors	Psychological Biological Developmental
Social factors	Friends Family Coworkers
Institutional factors	Companies Schools Health care facilities
Community factors	Organization of physical activity resources Activity-related events in place Safe walking, biking trails
Public policy	Tax breaks for healthy behaviors Laws protecting green space Better insurance rates for fit individuals

are more likely to lead to greater changes and longer-lasting maintenance of physical activity than those that don't (Sallis, Bauman, & Pratt, 1998). Furthermore, it is important to customize the program to the client's physical environment. For example, an outdoor walking program in an unsafe neighborhood or one with few sidewalks is not likely to be successful for many people. Table 3.2 provides some examples of environmental variables that affect physical activity behavior (Humpel, Owen, & Leslie, 2002).

Relapse Prevention Model

Although the relapse prevention model (figure 3.5) was originally developed to better understand people's difficulty with addictive behaviors, such as smoking and drinking (Marlatt & Gordon, 1985), it also has been useful in understanding and intervening to increase physical activity. The appeal of the relapse prevention model is that it is especially geared toward maintaining change over the long term. This is particularly important for a behavior such as physical activity because continuing to be active over time is necessary to maintain benefits. In fact, that is probably the biggest challenge in promoting physical activity—it does not do much good for people if they do not stick with it. Research has shown that men who were athletes in college but then stopped being active were no healthier than men who had never been active (Paffenbarger, Hyde, Wing, & Hsieh, 1986).

Programs based on the relapse prevention model help newly physically active people anticipate and plan for problems with sticking with their physical activity plans. Such problems include depression and anxiety, injury, social

TABLE 3.2 **Environmental Influences on Physical Activity**

Environmental influence	Examples
Accessibility of facilities	Bicycle paths Health clubs located nearby Walking paths Swimming pools
Opportunities for activities	Presence of sidewalks Home equipment Shops within walking distance Local fun runs held
Weather	Temperature Daylight changes Precipitation Wind
Safety	Crime rate Unattended dogs Street lighting Traffic levels
Aesthetics	Friendly neighborhood Enjoyable scenery Green space Hills, trees

Adapted from *American Journal of Preventive Medicine,* Vol 22, N. Humpel, N. Owen, and E. Leslie, "Environmental factors associated with adults' participation in physical activity," pgs. 188-191, with permission from Elsevier.

pressure, difficulties with family members or friends, limited social support, low motivation, time pressure, and bad weather (USDHHS, 1996). This theory suggests that it is first important to identify situations that place a person at high risk for not being physically active (e.g., putting in a lot of hours at work) and then to develop a game plan to avoid, or, if necessary, cope with, each of these situations (e.g., take two or three 10-minute walks as work breaks). If a person finds herself in a situation in which she is at risk for not being active but uses her skills to overcome the temptation to be sedentary, her self-efficacy is likely to increase. On the other hand, if she fails to be active, she is probably going to feel less confident in her abilities to handle similar situations in the future.

Another helpful aspect of the relapse prevention model is that it encourages people to make a distinction between a *lapse* (e.g., a few days of not being physically active) and a *relapse* (an extended period of no physical activity) so that they do not fall prey to the *abstinence violation effect*. This term refers to people's tendency to give up altogether when they have slipped. For example, a person who stops being active for a couple of weeks during a leisurely vacation may be disinclined to resume his activity program once he is home because he thinks, *What's the use? I'm out of the routine.* By acknowledging such a break in the physical activity habit as a normal but temporary occurrence, he will

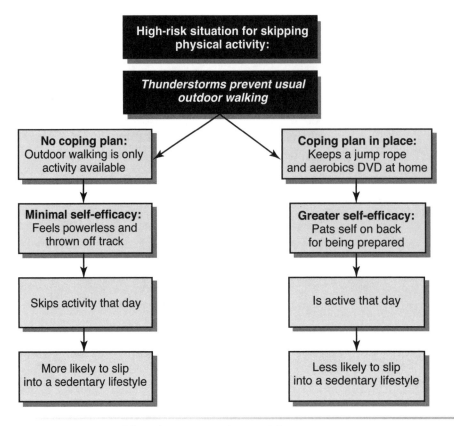

FIGURE 3.5   Diagram of the relapse prevention model.

Adapted, by permission, from G.A. Marlatt and J.R. Gordon, 1985, *Relapse prevention: Maintenance strategies in the treatment of addictive behaviors* (New York: Guilford Press), 38.

be more likely to tell himself, *Well, I had my break, but now it's time to start walking again.* It is inevitable that your client will experience lapses, but these periods do not necessarily need to result in a return to a sedentary lifestyle. Your job is to help your client plan for these potentially difficult situations.

Conclusion

You may have noticed that many of the ideas and program strategies discussed in this chapter are contained in the processes of change described in chapter 2. For example, the behavioral processes of rewarding yourself and committing yourself come from learning theory, social cognitive theory, and behavioral choice theory. The cognitive process of comprehending the benefits comes from behavioral choice theory, decision-making theory, and social cognitive theory. Increasing healthy opportunities is directly related to the environmental approach derived from the ecological model. The relapse prevention model is related to the processes of reminding yourself and substituting alternatives. Additionally, decisional balance, or the ratio of benefits to costs of physical

INTEGRATING OTHER PSYCHOLOGICAL THEORIES AND MODELS ▪ 33

activity (from decision-making theory), and self-efficacy (from social cognitive theory) have been shown to predict the stage of motivational readiness for physical activity (Marcus, Rakowski, et al., 1992; Marcus, Selby, Niaura, & Rossi, 1992) and physical activity behavior (Lewis et al., 2002). These examples highlight the transtheoretical nature of the processes of change. We hope that, after reading this chapter, you also recognize that physical activity is not easily or completely described by any one theory or model. Table 3.3 illustrates how ideas from several theories can be translated into change strategies. In turn, these strategies can be combined to produce a comprehensive program

TABLE 3.3   Promising Psychological Theories and Models for Promoting Physical Activity

Theory or model	Relevant ideas	Program strategies
Learning theory	• Shaping • Reinforcement • Stimulus control • Extrinsic vs. intrinsic rewards	• Self-monitoring • Goal setting • Rewards • Feedback
Decision-making theory	• Perceived benefits • Perceived barriers	• Decisional balance sheet • Removing barriers • Problem solving • Enhancing benefits
Behavioral choice theory	• Reinforcement • Benefits vs. barriers • Perceived choice • Availability of behavioral options	• Rewards • Decreasing sedentary options • Including client in planning and decision making • Increasing options for activity
Social cognitive theory	• Self-efficacy • Outcome expectations • Direct reinforcement • Observational learning	• Skill building • Setting achievable goals • Identifying benefits • Tangible rewards • Social support
Ecological model	• Personal skills • Institutional and community factors • Physical environment • Policies	• Self-management • Matching program to environmental opportunities • Altering physical environments to include more activity options
Relapse prevention model	• High-risk situations • Self-efficacy • Coping skills • Abstinence violation effect	• Planning • Confidence building • Problem solving • Identifying and changing negative thinking

that is likely to work. In other words, integrating the approaches suggested by multiple theories is more likely to lead to success than depending on any one model alone.

Behavioral intervention research on physical activity is a new area of scientific investigation, with very few studies conducted before 1990. Nonetheless, we have learned a great deal about physical activity behavior and how to help sedentary people become and stay more active. As a result, we can be confident that physical activity programs can succeed. Part II describes ways to implement the program strategies suggested by the models and theories described in this chapter within a stages of change framework.

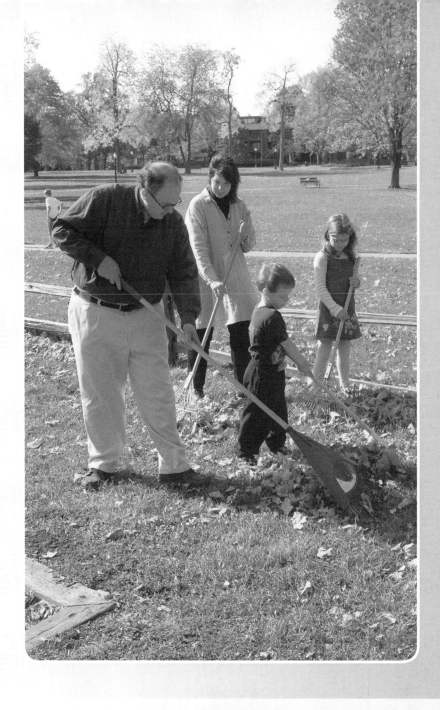

CHAPTER 4

Putting Theories to Work by Looking at Mediators of Change

Chapters 2 and 3 provided a description of some of the most promising psychological theories and models used to design successful physical activity programs. In this chapter we discuss constructs derived from these theories and models that are believed to produce, or *mediate,* behavior change. By becoming familiar with constructs derived from psychological and behavior change theory, you can incorporate strategies based on these constructs to build an effective physical activity program. We also include measures you can use to determine whether your intervention is affecting these constructs.

Consider Mediators of Physical Activity Behavior Change

When assessing the effectiveness of your interventions, you should consider not only measures of physical activity behavior or physical fitness but also changes in relevant psychological and behavioral mediators of physical activity behavior change. By paying attention to the parts of your program that were effective in helping your clients move toward a physically active lifestyle, you can learn what strategies work best for changing physical activity behaviors and get ideas for improving future programs (Baranowski, Anderson, & Carmack, 1998; Bauman, Sallis, Dzewaltowski, & Owen, 2002). In other words, is your intervention successful for the reasons suggested by the theory you used to design it? For instance, if encouraging your client to reward herself after reaching her activity goals appears to be partly responsible for your client's remaining active more days of the week, then you probably will want to incorporate that strategy into a program you design for someone else.

Assessing psychosocial constructs related to change becomes especially important as we work to discover what helps unmotivated people move toward considering a more active lifestyle. For people in stage 1 (not thinking about change) or stage 2 (thinking about change), it is probably unrealistic to expect to increase actual activity to the public health criterion level or to enhance physical fitness. Instead, a more realistic goal for these clients would be to promote change in factors that could lead to more physical activity down the road (e.g., identifying the pros of physical activity, enhanced self-efficacy). Helping a less motivated person to even start thinking about how his health and outlook might improve if he were to be more active should be considered a successful outcome. Therefore, learning what needs to happen within that person for change to occur (i.e., discovering the mediators) is well worth your time and effort as illustrated by the case example on page 37.

The theoretical model that serves as the basis for a program suggests which factors might be responsible for producing change in physical activity behavior. For example, a program based on social cognitive theory may focus on improving self-efficacy and outcome expectations for physical activity because changes in these factors are thought, in turn, to lead to more physical activity. When you hypothesize about possible mediators of your program's success,

Examining Mediators to Learn What Works

This case example demonstrates the usefulness of looking at change in the theoretical constructs used to design a physical activity intervention. In this program, two print-based programs were delivered to a community sample of sedentary but healthy adults (Marcus et al., 1998). One program was more theoretically based and used constructs derived from social cognitive theory and the transtheoretical model. In this program participants received motivationally tailored manuals along with individualized feedback reports on their progress in self-reported activity, stage of motivational readiness, self-efficacy, decisional balance, and use of processes of change (Jump Start: A Community-Based Program is described in more detail in chapter 5). The feedback reports were about four pages long and provided each participant with information regarding any personal improvements or declines in these areas and his or her standing in comparison with others who had become active.

The comparison program consisted of manuals from the American Heart Association (AHA) that were not tailored to participants in any way. These manuals were of similar length as the motivationally tailored manuals. The AHA manuals, although not personalized, provide excellent guidance on behavior change, advising starting gradually, setting goals, monitoring progress, and using other important behavioral processes of change. Materials were given at the start of the program and at 1, 3, and 6 months after the program began.

Both programs led to improvements in participants' physical activity levels. However, the group receiving the individually tailored feedback reported much more physical activity at 6 months than the comparison group did (Marcus et al., 1998). The investigators were interested in looking at possible changes in the theoretical constructs used in the individually tailored intervention to learn what aspects of this intervention made it more effective than the intervention that used standard print materials. What they found was that participants who had received the individually tailored intervention had greater improvement in their use of the behavioral processes of change and their self-efficacy for physical activity. Moreover, change in these constructs from baseline to 3 months predicted more minutes of physical activity at 6 months. The behavioral processes—specifically, reminding themselves (e.g., laying out exercise clothes to remind themselves to exercise later), committing themselves, rewarding themselves, and substituting alternatives—seemed to help participants in the individually tailored feedback group become more active. Only two behavioral processes (committing oneself and substituting alternatives) were related to improved physical activity levels in the comparison group. Therefore, providing people with individualized feedback about their ability to use behavioral processes appears to have encouraged them to use more of these processes than simply giving them a message about the processes. In turn, using more processes increases participants' chances of becoming active at recommended levels. This analysis of possible mediating constructs can be used to develop more effective print materials in future programs.

keep in mind that several mediators may be working at once (Baranowski et al., 1998). For example, self-efficacy, outcome expectations, and the use of several behavior change processes may mediate the results of your intervention. Therefore, it is wise to consider and measure several possible mediators. Combining theories (e.g., the transtheoretical model, social cognitive theory, decision-making theory) and building a program around several possible mediators (e.g., perceived benefits, behavioral processes of change, self-efficacy) are likely to make the program more successful as shown in table 4.1.

Factors That Enhance Physical Activity

In this section we describe some of the constructs derived from psychological theories and models that are believed to create change in physical activity behavior. As you will see, social cognitive theory (SCT) and the transtheoretical model (TTM) are the most commonly used theoretical frameworks in studies of physical activity mediators (Lewis et al., 2002).

Cognitive and Behavioral Processes of Change

According to the transtheoretical model, people use various cognitive and behavioral strategies and techniques to progress through the stages of motivational readiness for change (DiClemente et al., 1991; Prochaska & DiClemente, 1983). Studies have found that people in the later stages tend to use more of these processes than people in the earlier stages (Marcus, Rossi, Selby, Niaura, & Abrams, 1992). Accordingly, an increased use of behavioral processes has been shown to be significantly related to increases in physical activity behavior (Dunn et al., 1997; Lewis et al., 2002; Lewis et al., 2006; Nichols et al., 2000; Pinto, Lynn, Marcus, DePue, & Goldstein, 2001; Sallis, Calfas, Alcaraz, Gehrman, & Johnson, 1999). Studies of the cognitive processes serving as

TABLE 4.1   Using Theoretical Constructs to Change Physical Activity Motivation

Intervention		Change in mediators		Movement toward physical activity
Problem solving to decrease barriers		Perceiving more benefits		Shift from stage 2 to stage 3
Skills training	→	Use of more behavioral processes	→	More variety of activities attempted
Exercise role models		Greater self-efficacy		More minutes of physical activity

mediators of physical activity have been mixed, probably because people in the earlier stages of motivational readiness are not the ones participating in most physical activity interventions (Lewis et al., 2002); however, these processes are important for helping people in the earlier stages of motivational readiness move toward changing their actual physical activity behavior (Marcus, Rossi et al., 1992; Rosen, 2000). Examples of each of these processes of change are found in chapter 2.

Measuring Processes of Change A client's use of the processes of change for physical activity behavior can be measured with questionnaire 4.1 in appendix A, which we and our colleagues developed (Marcus, Rossi, Selby, Niaura, & Abrams, 1992). This questionnaire has been used in many exercise studies. When people's scores on these items increase, it is usually a good indicator that they are becoming more active (Dunn et al., 1997). The processes of change are the strategies and techniques people use to change their thinking and their behavior; your clients are therefore likely to increase their use of many of the processes of change long before they are meeting national guidelines for a physically active lifestyle.

You may want to have clients complete this questionnaire every 3 months so that you can learn whether they are making progress toward behavior change even if they are not meeting their specific physical activity goals. Recall that a person's stage of motivation for change when she first comes to see you has a great impact on how quickly she increases her use of the processes of change. The setting in which you work might also affect which processes of change increase first and how quickly the client puts them to use. For example, if you are a personal trainer at a health club, you are more likely to start working with clients on behavior change, and thus you are more likely to see increases in the behavioral processes of change. However, if you work at a community center, YMCA, or YWCA implementing a program such as the Active Living Program (Blair, Dunn, Marcus, Carpenter, & Jaret, 2001), you may see changes in your clients' cognitive processes before changes in their behavioral processes. Most published studies indicate that it is important for people to first increase their use of the cognitive processes and then of the behavioral processes. However, some studies indicate that the order is not important; people need to increase their use of all (or most) of the processes of change to become and stay regularly active (Marcus et al., 1992).

For each process of change, the average score can range from 1 to 5. Table 4.2 shows typical scores for the four items in each process group for people in each stage of motivational readiness for change. Use this as a guide for understanding where your client is in the change process and on which areas to focus to help her start and stick with a program of regular physical activity. If the survey results are similar on a number of processes, you can choose either a single process or, in collaboration with your client, several processes to work on.

Scoring Processes of Change   For each process, average the individual items by adding each group (shown in table 4.3) together and dividing by 4. Do not score an individual process if fewer than three items were answered.

TABLE 4.2   **Average Scores by Stage for the Processes of Change Questionnaire**

Process	Stage				
	1	2	3	4	5
Increasing knowledge	1.88	2.57	2.76	3.11	2.99
Being aware of risks	1.92	2.41	2.26	2.72	2.46
Caring about consequences to others	1.82	2.43	2.46	2.74	2.47
Comprehending benefits	2.14	3.13	3.22	3.66	3.28
Increasing healthy opportunities	2.14	2.55	2.75	2.81	2.79
Substituting alternatives	1.71	2.24	2.72	3.35	3.55
Enlisting social support	1.78	2.25	2.42	2.80	2.64
Rewarding oneself	1.52	2.25	2.54	2.99	3.01
Committing oneself	2.08	2.94	3.17	3.83	3.68
Reminding oneself	1.42	1.85	2.02	2.30	2.20

TABLE 4.3   **Grouping Related Items on the Processes of Change Questionnaire**

Process	Items
Increasing knowledge	5, 8, 17, 28
Being aware of risks	11, 12, 13, 14
Caring about consequences to others	30, 33, 34, 37
Comprehending benefits	15, 31, 35, 38
Increasing healthy opportunities	10, 22, 32, 36
Substituting alternatives	1, 21, 39, 40
Enlisting social support	16, 19, 24, 25
Rewarding oneself	7, 18, 20, 23
Committing oneself	2, 4, 6, 27
Reminding oneself	3, 9, 26, 29

Self-Efficacy

Self-efficacy refers to confidence in one's ability to perform specific behaviors in specific situations (Bandura, 1986, 1997). For example, in many parts of the United States, people often have higher self-efficacy (i.e., feel very self-confident) regarding their ability to maintain a walking program during the spring and summer months but do not see themselves keeping up with their activity in the cold, snowy winter. This is not surprising, given that maintaining some type of physical activity in the winter often requires a new set of behaviors such as going to an indoor facility or learning how to dress appropriately for activity in cold weather. Another example illustrates how self-efficacy is also behavior specific. Many people have a high level of self-efficacy for some types of physical activity such as brisk walking but feel less confident in their ability to incorporate additional types of activity (e.g., swimming) that would be beneficial for increasing variety and reducing the risks of boredom and overuse injuries. Some studies have investigated self-efficacy for physical activity across various situations, such as during vacation, when injured, and during bad weather (Marcus, Selby, Niaura, & Rossi, 1992). Others have looked at self-efficacy for various components of being physically active, such as making time for activity and sticking to it (Sallis, Pinski, Grossman, Patterson, & Nader, 1988).

According to social cognitive theory, self-efficacy is the most important mediator of behavior change (Bandura, 1986, 1997), and this has been demonstrated across studies looking at mediating constructs of successful interventions (Brassington, Atienza, Perczek, DiLorenzo, & King, 2002; Lewis et al., 2002). In other words, improved self-efficacy leads to higher levels of physical activity at some later time (usually measured 3 to 6 months after the start of the program).

Measuring Self-Efficacy   We recommend measuring physical activity–specific self-efficacy with questionnaire 4.2 in appendix A, which we and our colleagues developed (Marcus, Selby, Niaura, & Rossi, 1992). This brief, five-item questionnaire measures the major components of self-efficacy and has been used in many physical activity studies. People's self-efficacy scores almost always increase as they become more active. As with the processes of change questionnaire, we encourage you to administer the self-efficacy questionnaire to your clients every 3 months. If a client's score on this measure is not increasing, this is a red flag; you need to discuss this lack of self-efficacy with him because his belief that he cannot succeed with physical activity does not bode well for his becoming and staying active for life.

Scoring Self-Efficacy   Calculate the score on the self-efficacy questionnaire by computing the average of all five items for each client. If any of the items are unanswered, have the client fill them in before scoring. A higher score on this measure indicates greater self-efficacy. Increased self-efficacy is important for a person to adopt and maintain a program of regular physical activity.

Social Support

Social support is believed to be another strong mediator of behavior change (Lewis et al., 2002; Sarason & Sarason, 1985). The four types of social support are instrumental, informational, emotional, and appraising (Cohen, Mermelstein, Kamarck, & Hoberman, 1985). *Instrumental* support involves giving another person something tangible to encourage behavior change. Examples of instrumental support are giving a person a ride to an exercise facility or giving a spouse a treadmill as a birthday gift. *Informational* social support involves helping a person make behavior changes by providing relevant information. For example, you might tell a friend about an upcoming fun run or talk to your sister about the processes you use to keep yourself motivated. *Emotional* support is letting another person know that you care about him and how he is doing in his attempt to change his behavior. When you call a friend or family member to see how he is faring with his attempt to be active for 20 minutes each day, you are offering emotional support. Finally, the fourth type of social support, *appraising,* involves providing feedback and encouragement to someone learning a new physical activity skill. An aerobics instructor provides this type of support when she tells a class participant that she has noticed her improvement over the last few weeks. As these examples illustrate, social support can come from many sources, such as family members, friends, coworkers, exercise instructors, and other participants in an exercise class (Miller, Steart, Trost, & Brown, 2002; Stoddard, Palombo, Troped, Sorensen, & Will, 2004; USDHHS, 1996).

Physical activity research has looked at both general social support and social support specific to physical activity. A study comparing the two found that they are quite distinct (Sallis et al., 1987). A woman may believe that she has good social support in most areas of her life (e.g., a husband who helps with household responsibilities, friends and family members with whom she feels comfortable sharing her feelings and concerns) yet believe that few people share her interest in physical activity, can give advice about being physically active, or will help with child care responsibilities so that she can make the time for physical activity. In a program designed to help sedentary mothers of young children increase their physical activity, increased support from the children's fathers was associated with the mothers' ability to become more physically active (Miller, Trost, & Brown, 2006).

Measuring Social Support for Physical Activity   We recommend using a questionnaire that was developed specifically to measure physical activity–related social support from family and friends (questionnaire 4.3 in appendix A) (Sallis et al., 1987). The client should answer each question for both family and friends (there is a separate column to check for each). This instrument asks about exercise-related support obtained in the last 3 months, so you may want to administer it at 3-month intervals to detect any changes. If your client receives a low score for social support from either friends or family, you may want to suggest some strategies for enhancing social support from these people (e.g., providing child care if needed or becoming an activity partner) because higher scores are associated with greater success in changing health habits and with better physical activity adherence (Courneya & McAuley, 1995; Miller et al., 2002; Oka, King, & Young, 1995; Sallis et al., 1987).

Scoring Social Support for Physical Activity   To score the measure for social support for physical activity, first invert the responses to questions 7 and 8 (1 = 5, 2 = 4, 3 = 3, 4 = 2, 5 = 1). Then sum all the items for family support and all the items for friend support separately. Higher scores reflect more perceived social support from these people.

Decisional Balance

Decisional balance—the ratio of perceived benefits to barriers of change—comes from Janis and Mann's (1977) decision-making theory. With regard to physical activity behavior change, decisional balance refers to a person's perception of the benefits of physical activity compared to its negative aspects (Janis & Mann, 1977; Marcus, Rakowski, & Rossi, 1992). Some people view physical activity in a positive light, whereas others focus more on its downside. Some perceived barriers are environmental, such as bad weather, an unsafe neighborhood for walking, and a lack of available parks, sidewalks, and bicycle paths. Other barriers are more personal, such as believing you do not have enough time or energy to be physically active after work. Fear of becoming injured, lack of motivation, and unhelpful friends or family members are other examples of personal barriers.

Differences in decisional balance tend to correspond to the various stages of motivational readiness. People in stage 1 (not thinking about change) perceive more barriers to than benefits of change, whereas those in the later stages perceive more benefits than barriers (Marcus & Owen, 1992; Marcus, Rakowski, & Rossi, 1992). Research has shown that for people to become more active, they need to see lots of benefits and not too many barriers to becoming more active. Over time, people tend to see more benefits of than barriers to physical activity, and that is important to keeping them active over the long term. Indeed, higher scores on the decisional balance measure (i.e., viewing physical activity in a more positive light than a negative one) have been shown to predict increases in physical activity behavior (Dunn et al., 1997; Pinto et al., 2001).

Measuring Decisional Balance   We recommend using the decisional balance questionnaire (questionnaire 4.4 in appendix A) that we and our colleagues developed (Marcus, Rakowski, & Rossi, 1992) to measure physical activity decision making. This questionnaire measures a client's perceived benefits of and barriers to physical activity.

Scoring Decisional Balance   Compute the averages of the 10 pro items and of the 6 con items.

- ▪ Pros = (item 1 + item 2 + item 4 + item 5 + item 6 + item 8 + item 9 + item 10 + item 12 + item 14) / 10
- ▪ Cons = (item 3 + item 7 + item 11 + item 13 + item 15 + item 16) / 6

The difference in the averages (i.e., pros minus cons) is the decisional balance score. Decisional balance scores greater than 0 indicate that your client sees more benefits of than barriers to being active. The larger the score, the more benefits your client sees relative to barriers. A score less than 0 indicates that your client sees more barriers to than benefits of being physically active. The larger the negative score, the more barriers your client sees relative to benefits. It is important to help your client see both more benefits of and fewer barriers to physical activity. If your program is successful, you will likely see scores on this questionnaire move from negative to positive and then continue to rise.

Outcome Expectations

Outcome expectations refers to the value a person places on the outcomes or consequences he believes will occur as a result of being physically active. Researchers have found that people with greater outcome expectations for exercise are more likely to adopt and maintain regular physical activity (Brassington et al., 2002; Hallam & Petosa, 1998). Some of these outcomes occur immediately after being active, such as feeling energized. Other outcomes require being physically active for some time, such as losing weight or having more muscle tone. Specific outcome expectations that have been used to predict physical activity behavior include health benefits, improved body image, and psychological benefits such as stress reduction (Steinhardt & Dishman,1989).

Measuring Outcome Expectations   The brief Outcome Expectations for Exercise (OEE) scale (Resnick, Zimmerman, Orwig, Furstenberg, & Magaziner, 2000) can be used to measure your clients' expected benefits from activity (see questionnaire 4.5 in appendix A). This scale asks about both the physical and mental benefits expected. If you find that your client has low expectations for physical activity, you should work with her to identify some benefits she is likely to experience as a result of her activity. Doing so may help strengthen her outcome expectations, which in turn may improve her physical activity behavior.

Scoring Outcome Expectations   This measure is scored by summing the ratings for all the items and dividing by 9 to get the average of all 9 items. Scores can range from 1 to 5, with 1 indicating low outcome expectations for exercise and 5 suggesting high outcome expectations. Although the measure is used to obtain an overall score for outcome expectations, you can look at your client's scores on the individual items to determine the areas in which she believes she is less likely to benefit. Then you can focus on improving these areas.

Enjoyment

People who say they enjoy physical activity tend to be the ones who become and stay active (Wankel, 1993). Indeed, enjoyment of physical activity is associated with stage of motivational readiness for change, adherence to structured exercise programs, and increased levels of physical activity behavior (Leslie et al., 1999; Rovniak, Anderson, Winett, & Stephens, 2002; Stevens, Lemmink, de Greef, & Rispens, 2000; Williams, Papandonatos, Napolitano, & Lewis, 2006; USDHHS, 1996). Although enjoyment of physical activity is not directly related to any specific theory, some have argued that it can be conceptualized as a type of outcome expectancy since enjoyment has been assumed to be related to a person's willingness to be active (Williams, Anderson, & Winett, 2005). Therefore, it follows that if we can help a client enjoy physical activity more, that client is more likely to be active later on. This is supported by a recent study that found that a school-based intervention enhanced adolescent girls' enjoyment of physical activity, which in turn led to increased physical activity behavior (Dishman et al., 2005).

Measuring Physical Activity Enjoyment   The Physical Activity Enjoyment Scale (PACES; see questionnaire 4.6 in appendix A) is an 18-item measure that can be used to determine how enjoyable your client finds exercise. The developers of this measure say that it can be used for any physical activity (Kendzierski & DeCarlo, 1991). You can help clients who score low on this measure to find activities that are more pleasurable, or you can adjust their activities so they are less unpleasant (e.g., suggest they listen to music while being active, engage in a moderate-intensity activity rather than a vigorous one, or talk to a partner during activity).

Scoring Physical Activity Enjoyment   For items 1, 4, 5, 7, 9, 10, 11, 13, 14, 16, and 17, assign point values as follows:

If the client answered

1, give a score of 7   5, give a score of 3

2, give a score of 6   6, give a score of 2

3, give a score of 5   7, give a score of 1

4, give a score of 4

Then add all the items. Higher scores reflect greater enjoyment from physical activity. You can give this measure to your client periodically (e.g., every month or two) to see whether his enjoyment increases as he becomes more skilled and physically fit over time. Or you can have your client complete this questionnaire after you have made some suggestions for making physical activity more fun and he has had a chance to try out your ideas. This can be a way of determining what makes activity more pleasurable for your client.

Unlock the "Black Box"

Although many physical activity programs are based on psychological theories and models, few studies test to see whether the program changed the theoretical constructs used to design the program (Baranowski et al., 1998; Lewis et al., 2002). To do this, researchers first must determine whether the program changed possible mediators. For example, did a program based on social cognitive theory, which emphasizes self-efficacy, really help participants become more confident in their ability to become and stay active, and did a change in self-efficacy lead to participants' actually becoming more physically active? Furthermore, interventions are sometimes more effective for some populations and less effective for others. These concepts are explained in more detail in the sidebar, "Learning How it Works."

LEARNING HOW IT WORKS

Moderators Versus Mediators

If you are interested in learning more about testing the theories you use to design your intervention, you should understand what is meant by the terms *mediator* and *moderator*. Although the terms are often used interchangeably in the literature, the function of a moderator is quite different from that of a mediator (Baron & Kenny, 1986; Bauman et al., 2002). Let us briefly explain.

Moderators: A moderator is a factor used to divide participants into subgroups for whom the intervention works differently (Baron & Kenny, 1986; Bauman et al., 2002). For example, one study found that a motivationally tailored intervention was more effective for people in the earlier stages of motivational readiness (i.e., stage 1, not thinking about change, and stage 2, thinking about change) compared to a program that was not motivationally tailored. However, both interventions were equally effective for people who were in stage 3 (doing some activity) (Marcus et al., 1998). In this case, stage of motivational readiness was a moderator of the tailored intervention's effectiveness. Personal factors such as age, gender, health status, mood, and socioeconomic status may be related to the effectiveness of a program and therefore may serve as moderators. Aspects of participants' physical environment (e.g., crime rate, availability of sidewalks, green space, and level of traffic congestion) may also serve as moderators that determine subgroups for whom a given intervention may be more or less effective (King, Stokols, Talin, Brassington, & Killingsworth, 2002). Moderators tell us *who* will benefit most from a program, but they do not tell us *how* the intervention works. To determine this, we look at factors that change as a result of a program: the mediators.

Mediators: In contrast to many moderators (e.g., age, gender), a mediator is always a factor that can help a given client personally change. A mediator represents the mechanism by which the intervention is believed to influence physical activity behavior (Baron & Kenny, 1986; Bauman et al., 2002). Again, let us illustrate with an example. You might design a program based on the decision-making theory that attempts to help clients identify more benefits of becoming active and reduce the number of excuses (barriers) they make for being inactive. The theory is based on the assumption that if your clients associate more positives and fewer negatives with physical activity, they will be more likely to become and stay physically active. In this example, perceptions of positive and negative aspects of physical activity are believed to be mediators of behavior change. Prior to starting your program, you measure perceived benefits and perceived barriers and find that your clients do indeed see more barriers than benefits. After you complete your intervention and find that your clients have become more active, you decide to again measure their perceived benefits and barriers. If you find that your clients now see more benefits of being active and identify fewer excuses for staying sedentary, you have some evidence that your intervention's ability to improve decisional balance (i.e., ratio of perceived benefits to barriers; see chapter 3) helped your clients to become more active. At a higher level of sophistication, you might actually track changes in perceived benefits and perceived obstacles by repeated measurement of these variables to see whether changes occur first in these mediators prior to increases in physical activity behavior. If so, you will have demonstrated that changes in mediating variables in turn led to increases in physical activity. To learn more about various influences on physical activity, you can refer to Bauman, Sallis, Dzewaltowski, and Owen (1992), and for a review of psychosocial mediators tested in various interventions, to Lewis et al. (2002).

Conclusion

Several untested mediators may warrant further attention. For example, would a program that helps people make changes in their environment (e.g., moving the treadmill out of the spare bedroom and into the main living area or creating exercise space in the workplace) help them become more active? Would helping a client view her physical appearance (i.e., body image) more positively influence her activity levels down the road because she is less embarrassed to be seen exercising? Would including a client's family and friends in the program help that client to be more active? Considering factors such as these, addressing them in your program, and then measuring them to see whether they change as a result of your program can help to open up the "black box" of changing physical activity behavior. The chapters in part II discuss strategies for influencing physical activity mediators.

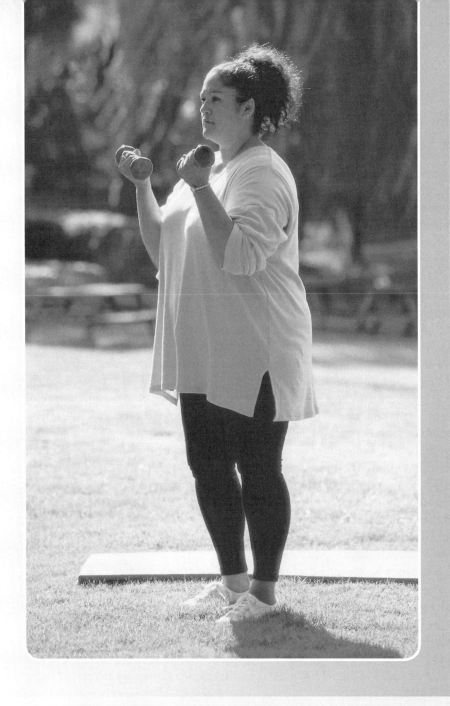

CHAPTER 5

Using the Stages Model for Successful Physical Activity Interventions

Client treatment matching is a concept that has been popular for years in the psychotherapy field. The idea that programs should be matched to the specific characteristics and needs of the client has also gained popularity in programs for quitting smoking and weight loss. However, we are just beginning to learn how to match physical activity programs to our target audiences. This concept has been slow to reach the arena of exercise and physical activity programs in part because leading a sedentary lifestyle has only recently begun to receive national recognition as a significant public health problem (Fletcher et al., 1992; Haskell et al., 2007; Pate et al., 1995; USDHHS, 1996, 2000). Most urban and some rural communities have a large number of gyms, community exercise programs, and health clubs, so resources are available for most people to exercise. Nevertheless, much of our population is sedentary, and most people who start an exercise program do not stick with it over the long term (Dishman, 1994; Marcus et al., 2000). Therefore, the time seems right to consider client program matching for the promotion of physical activity.

The stages of motivational readiness for change model is founded on the idea that people differ in their levels of readiness to change their behavior. Therefore, programs need to use differing strategies and techniques to bring about desired behavior changes. For example, the program goal for a client starting in stage 1 (not thinking about change) could be to help the client to begin to think about change by reading articles about the health, body image, and self-esteem benefits of physical activity and perhaps by taking a couple of 10-minute walks during the course of a week. In contrast, the goal of a program for a client in stage 3 (doing some physical activity) might be helping the client to take daily 10-minute walks and then building up to 30-minute walks on at least 5 days of the week.

In this chapter we describe a few physical activity programs that have used the stages of change model. Earlier programs were able to attract people who were already physically active but had a harder time reaching those who were not. Part of the reason for this may have been the program names. Not surprisingly, a program called Get Fit recruited people who were already active and wanted to become more fit or to maintain their fitness. Programs targeted at people in stage 2 have used names such as Imagine Action or Jump Start to Health.

Imagine Action: A Community-Based Program

The Imagine Action campaign was a community-wide physical activity program (Marcus et al., 1992). Participants were adults who enrolled through their workplaces or in response to advertisements. Potential participants received a description of the program with a letter explaining that if they were inactive or having difficulty staying active, this program was designed for them. Respondents provided information about their activity level, name, address, sex, and birth date and were given a free T-shirt for enrolling. On average, participants were 42 years old, and 77% were women. At baseline, 39% were in stage 2 (thinking about change), 37% were in stage 3 (doing some physical activity), and 24% were in stage 4 (doing enough physical activity).

The program lasted 6 weeks and consisted of stage-matched self-help materials, a resource manual, and weekly fun walks and activity nights. The stage-matched materials were based on the exercise-adherence literature and informed by the stages of motivational readiness for change model, social cognitive theory, and decision-making theory. The manual for those in stage 2, called *What's in It for You,* included information on increasing lifestyle physical activity (e.g., taking the stairs instead of the elevator, parking at the far end of the parking lot), considering the benefits of (e.g., weight control) and barriers to (e.g., activity takes too much time) becoming more active, the social benefits of activity (e.g., meeting people in a class, walking with a friend), and rewarding oneself for increasing activity (e.g., buying a new CD as a reward for increasing from one to two walks per week).

The self-help manual for those in stage 3 was called *Ready for Action* because this group was participating in some activity but less than the goal of 30 minutes of moderate-intensity activity daily or 20 minutes of vigorous activity three to five times per week. This manual addressed the barriers to and benefits of physical activity, setting short-term activity goals (e.g., making time for a daily walk) and longer-term activity goals (e.g., walking for 30 minutes five times per week), rewarding oneself for activity, time management to fit activity into a busy schedule (e.g., walking on treadmill while watching the news on television), and details on developing a walking program.

The self-help manual for those in stage 4 was called *Keep It Going,* because these people had been regularly active only for a short time and thus were at risk for relapse to stage 3. This manual focused on troubleshooting situations that might lead to relapse (e.g., illness, injury, boredom), goal setting, rewarding oneself (both internal rewards such as self-praise and external rewards such as buying oneself flowers), cross-training to prevent boredom, avoiding injury, and gaining social support (e.g., finding people with whom to be active or who support an active lifestyle).

The resource manual described a wide variety of free and low-cost light-intensity, moderate-intensity, and vigorous physical activity options in the local community. The organized physical activity options included fun walks and appropriate free classes at local facilities, such as low-impact aerobics and volleyball for people who have never played.

Following the program, 30% of those in stage 2 and 61% of those in stage 3 at baseline progressed to stage 4 (doing enough physical activity), and an additional 31% who had been in stage 2 progressed to stage 3. Only 4% of those in stage 3 and 9% of those in stage 4 at the baseline slipped back to an earlier stage of motivational readiness. These findings demonstrate that a low-cost, relatively low-intensity program can produce important changes in physical activity.

Jump Start to Health: A Workplace-Based Study

The Jump Start to Health study examined the usefulness of a stage-matched physical activity program in the workplace for healthy, sedentary employees (Marcus, Emmons, et al., 1998). Employees were recruited through signs about the study placed around the workplace. Participating employees were placed at random in either a stage-matched self-help program or a non-stage-matched self-help program. The programs consisted of print materials delivered at the beginning of the study and 1 month later. Baseline stage of readiness and other information about physical activity habits were determined by having employees fill out a series of questionnaires in a private area at each participating workplace. At most of the workplaces, employees were given time off from work to fill out the questionnaires. At some workplaces, employees needed to use break time, lunchtime, or time after work. Free popcorn and beverages were available to employees who filled out questionnaires. Additionally, each employee who participated received a $1 Rhode Island State lottery ticket.

At the beginning of the study, people in the stage-matched group received manuals specifically tailored to their stage of motivational readiness for change (figure 5.1). One month later, these people received the manual matched to their current stage plus the manual for the next stage. The manual for those in stage 1 (not thinking about change), titled *Do I Need This?*, focused on increasing awareness of the benefits of activity and the barriers that prevented people from being active. Specific suggestions for starting an exercise routine were not provided in this manual. The manual for those thinking about change (stage 2), titled *Try It, You'll Like It,* included a discussion of the reasons to stay inactive versus the reasons to become more active, learning to reward oneself, and setting realistic goals.

For those in stage 3 (doing some physical activity), *I'm on My Way* reviewed the benefits of activity, goal setting, and tips on safe and enjoyable activities, and addressed obstacles to regular activity (e.g., lack of time, feeling too tired). *Keep It Going* provided information for those in stage 4 (doing enough physical activity) on the benefits of regular activity, staying motivated, rewarding oneself, enhancing confidence about being active, and overcoming obstacles. For those in stage 5 (making physical activity a habit), *I Won't Stop Now* emphasized the benefits of regular activity, avoiding injuries, setting goals, varying activities, rewarding oneself, and planning ahead. (These manuals can be ordered by calling 1-401-793-8081 or sending an e-mail to LSExercise@lifespan.org.)

People in the non-stage-matched group received American Heart Association manuals (AHA, 1984a, 1984b, 1984c, 1984d, 1989). These print materials were selected as a comparison intervention because they are of excellent quality and readily available.

An examination of participants' responses to questionnaires at the beginning of the program and 3 months later revealed that more subjects in the stage-

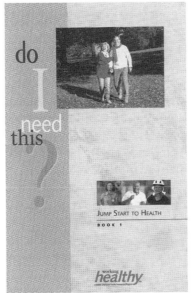
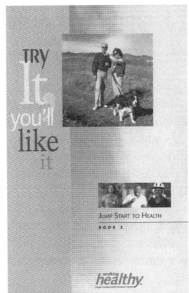
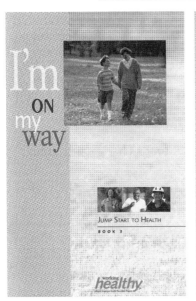
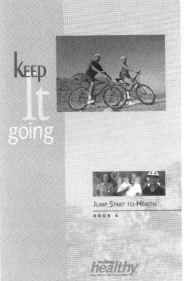
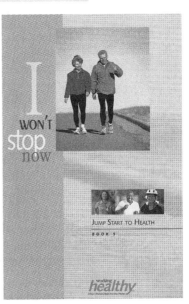

FIGURE 5.1 Manuals tailored to the various stages of motivational readiness for physical activity behavior change.

matched group than in the non-stage-matched group became more active (37% versus 27%). The stage-matched approach was particularly effective for those who entered the program in stage 1, 2, or 3, which is noteworthy because these are the types of people who are most likely to be your clients.

Jump Start: A Community-Based Study

A community-based study compared a standard print-based program (AHA 1984a, 1984b, 1984c, 1984d, 1989) to a stage-matched print program that also provided individualized feedback to participants each time they filled out a questionnaire about their physical activity behavior (Marcus, Bock, et al., 1998). The goal was to give participants tailored comparisons between their own behaviors and those of other participants who had been successful. Additionally, feedback informed participants about how they had changed since the last time they filled out the questionnaires so that they understood whether they were moving forward, sliding backward, or doing about the same on a variety of strategies and techniques shown to be important for becoming long-term physically active people.

Following are examples of two types of such feedback. The first example gives a comparison between the individual and other successful participants:

> Your answers show that you are well aware of the benefits of regular exercise. This is something that you have in common with others in the program who have also made good progress. Because you already do some exercise, it's now important for you to gradually become more active and make exercise a more frequent and consistent part of your life. Now is the time to think about the things that could stop you from exercising regularly. Being prepared for the problems you may encounter is a big help in sticking to an exercise program. You will be better prepared to overcome obstacles by thinking about the kinds of thoughts and activities that will help you remain active during difficult periods.

This is an example of feedback regarding the individual's change since the prior assessment:

> Your answers show that since we last heard from you, you have been taking more responsibility for your own health and well-being. You are also becoming more aware of the importance of believing in yourself and your ability to remain active. That's great! However, you are thinking a bit less about these issues than others who have succeeded in becoming and staying active.

> To make more progress, try making a commitment to being more active. Think about the things you have done before, achievements you have made, goals you have reached. Try setting small goals for yourself that you know you can meet, such as going for a short walk or adding a few extra minutes of activity into each day. This will help you strengthen your sense of accomplishment.

The individualized feedback concerned the topics of motivation, cognitive and behavioral strategies for becoming more active, barriers to and benefits from exercise, self-efficacy, and minutes of physical activity per week. Participants received printed reports and stage-matched manuals at the beginning of the program when they were first assessed by questionnaire and 1, 3, and 6 months later.

Results showed that those who received the individualized program were more likely to achieve recommended levels of physical activity (accumulating at least 30 minutes of physical activity per day at least 5 days per week) and were more likely to maintain that activity through a 12-month follow-up period than were participants who were given standard materials promoting physical activity (Bock, Marcus, Pinto, & Forsyth, 2001; Marcus, Bock, et al., 1998). Thus, this study shows that using materials matched to each participant's specific characteristics is helpful in increasing physical activity.

Project Active: A Community-Based Study

Project Active also was based on the stages of motivational readiness for change model; it had the benefit of following participants for 18 months after the initial phase of the program (Dunn et al., 1999). Project Active was a 2-year study that compared a lifestyle physical activity program (which encouraged participants to fit in 10-minute walks whenever they could) with a structured exercise program (which offered free membership at a beautiful gym). This study was conducted to compare the physical and psychological benefits of the lifestyle approach with those of a more traditional, structured exercise program in which it is more difficult to take into account an individual's motivation for change, unique barriers, and the like.

The lifestyle group members met for hour-long behaviorally oriented meetings each week that gradually decreased in frequency after the first 4 months of the program. Specific topics that were discussed are given in chapter 8; they included the following:

- Setting realistic goals for activity
- Finding someone to support you so that you can be active
- Learning how to reward yourself for being active

The structured-group participants were given a 6-month membership to a fitness center and met with an exercise trainer who provided the type of support offered in many health clubs. These participants gradually increased their workouts to 5 days a week for at least 30 minutes of duration.

After the 6-month program, both groups were much more active than at the beginning of the study (Dunn et al., 1998). Additionally, 30% of participants were meeting the CDC/ACSM recommendations of participating in at least 30 minutes of moderate-intensity physical activity at least 5 days per week (compared to none at the beginning of the study). After the entire 2-year study period, both groups still showed improvements in energy expenditure and cardiorespiratory fitness compared with the beginning of the program (Dunn et al., 1999). Thus, regardless of the setting in which you work, we encourage you to think broadly about the type of activity to encourage. The lifestyle approach may work best for many people, especially those starting out in stage 1 or 2. The curriculum used for Project Active, titled *Active Living Every Day*, is available through Human Kinetics. This workbook contains information that your client can use on her own or with your assistance. Topics such as setting goals, enlisting support, gaining confidence, and rewarding yourself are included.

Project STRIDE: A Community-Based Study

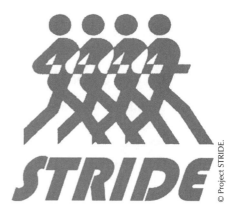
© Project STRIDE.

Given that only 32% of Americans meet physical activity recommendations, there is a need to develop effective, evidence-based interventions to promote physical activity that can be made widely available (Barnes & Schoenborn, 2003). Thus, we sought to test two delivery channels, telephone and print, to determine whether one was more effective than the other to promote physical activity among healthy, sedentary adults. Both intervention arms were guided by a motivationally tailored, theoretically driven computer expert system covering topics similar to the ones discussed in the stage-based manuals used in the Jump Start study described earlier. Additionally, participants filled out questionnaires on a monthly basis during the first 6 months of the program and bimonthly during the second 6 months of the program to provide the information needed to tailor their print or telephone feedback (Marcus, Napolitano, Lewis, et al., 2007). At 6 months, participants in both the telephone and print arms significantly increased their minutes of moderate-intensity physical activity compared to controls, with no differences between the intervention arms (mean minutes for print = 129.49 and for phone = 123.32). At 12 months, print participants reported a significantly greater number of moderate-intensity minutes than both telephone and control participants (mean minutes for print = 162.37 and for phone = 100.59) (Marcus, Napolitano, King, et al., 2007). Results suggest that both telephone and print interventions enhance the adoption of physical activity among sedentary adults; however, print interventions may be particularly effective in maintaining physical activity in the longer term.

Step Into Motion: A Community-Based Study

Because over two-thirds of Americans access the Internet, it may be an important channel for reaching the large population of sedentary people (Madden, 2006). Step Into Motion, a study based on the transtheoretical model, tested a Web-based version of the protocol used in Project STRIDE (Marcus, Lewis, et al., 2007b). The sample consisted of mostly women (84.2%) and Caucasian individuals (76.4%) who reported exercising an average of 21 minutes per week at baseline. In this study 44.4% of the participants who received the tailored Internet-based intervention achieved the public health recommended levels of physical activity

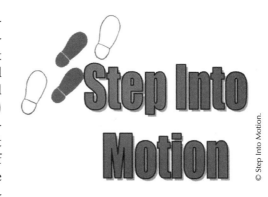

© Step Into Motion.

at 6 months (mean minutes per week = 161.4), and 39.5% achieved these levels at 12 months (mean minutes per week = 123.2). This is an important finding considering that this Internet-based intervention was technologically restricted to properly match and compare it to our print-based intervention (e.g., no chat rooms, no blogs, limited interactivity) (Marcus, Lewis, et al., 2007a). Thus, we have found the Internet to be a viable tool that can be used to increase physical activity among sedentary, healthy adults. However, to date, Internet interventions designed to promote physical activity have not taken full advantage of rapidly improving Web-based features such as blogs, chat rooms, and polls. Additional research is needed to examine how these components of the Internet can more effectively help people adopt and maintain physical activity behavior.

Conclusion

Overall, the studies described in this chapter suggest that using a stage-matched approach helps people progress toward more active lifestyles. These studies also demonstrate that matching interventions to participants' levels of motivational readiness is a more effective approach than using a one-treatment-fits-all approach in which all people receive the same information regardless of their motivation to change their activity levels. Personalizing information to the individual was found to be important. In the setting in which you work, accomplishing this personalization may be more or less feasible, but it is nonetheless important.

Another important finding of these studies is that effective programs need not be the traditional gym-based ones with which you may be quite familiar. Lifestyle activity programs are also quite effective in helping your clients achieve the improvements in health and fitness they want.

Here ends part I, in which we focused on the theoretical background and tools for measuring motivational readiness for change. In part II we focus on applying the stages of motivational readiness for change model in individual, group, work, and community settings.

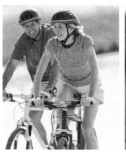
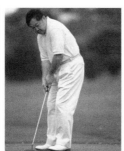
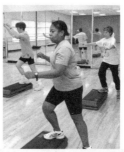
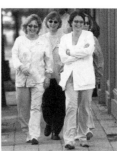
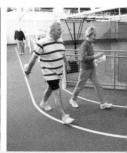

Applications

In part II we describe the assessment of patterns of physical activity and physical fitness, and we also examine applications of the stages of motivational readiness for change model to various settings. We explain how to measure your clients' physical activity patterns and physical fitness as well as discuss how to apply the stages of the motivational readiness for change model to individual, group, work site, and community settings. Then we discuss how you can apply these concepts to specific populations with whom you are working. Within this section we also provide exercises and worksheets that you can use in your physical activity programs and case studies that we hope will give you creative ideas of how you might use the information presented.

PART

two

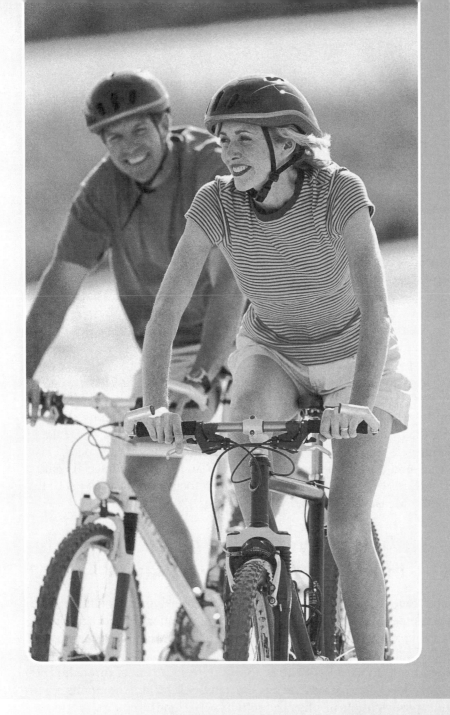

CHAPTER 6

Assessing Physical Activity Patterns and Physical Fitness

It is important for your clients to keep track of their participation in physical activity so that you know exactly what they are doing and can help them develop short- and long-term plans to reach their goals. Understanding patterns of behavior is an important first step for developing a plan to promote increases in physical activity behavior. Once you understand how a client spends his time, you can begin to think of creative options to help him fit in some physical activity at times when he has been doing none and more activity at times when he has been doing a little.

In this chapter we describe a variety of ways to track activity patterns and help clients determine the intensity of their physical activity. We discuss the use of the stages of change questionnaire, introduced in chapter 2 (see questionnaire 2.1 in appendix A), to examine patterns of physical activity behavior. We describe a system for tracking 10- and 30-minute bouts of light, moderate, and vigorous activity and another for recording everything done during the day and whether these activities are forms of physical activity. Next we introduce the idea of tracking physical activity habits with a step counter. We describe using resting heart rate and time to walk half a mile (0.8 km) to measure physical fitness. We conclude by mentioning strategies for using these tools with more than one person at a time. For more details about strategies for measuring physical activity, see the 1997 special issue of *Medicine and Science in Sports and Exercise* and the 2000 special issue of *Research Quarterly for Exercise and Sport,* which focus on this topic ("A Collection," 1997; "Measurement of Physical Activity," 2000).

Discovering Patterns of Physical Activity Behavior

In chapter 2 we discussed determining a client's stage of motivational readiness for change. Although the stages of change questionnaire (questionnaire 2.1 in appendix A) does not allow you to learn about exact patterns of physical activity, such as the times of day the person was active or whether she performed her activity all at once or in multiple short bouts throughout the day, it does allow you to assess her current activity level and intentions regarding future participation in physical activity. This questionnaire works well as a complement to other measures that provide detailed information about the number of minutes of physical activity per day and the types of activity performed. If global patterns of behavior and intention are most important in the setting in which you work, the stages of change questionnaire might be sufficient for your goals. This questionnaire is very brief, and studies have shown that scores on this measure correspond well with actual minutes of physical activity (Marcus & Simkin, 1993).

Determining Intensity Level

We currently know the health benefits associated with moderate- and vigorous-intensity activity; however, we do not know about the health benefits associated with light activity. Therefore, one of your goals when working with clients is to help them understand the intensity in which they need to perform their physical activity to achieve health benefits. Some clients will be surprised to learn that they can gain health benefits from moderate-intensity endeavors such as raking leaves or dancing with their kids. Others will be surprised that they need to work a little harder when they take the dog for a walk if they want to truly improve their mental and physical health. Table 6.1 shows categories of activities and examples of moderate-intensity and vigorous-intensity activities in each category. To help a client determine whether a given physical activity is of light, moderate, or vigorous intensity for him, you can use one of the methods discussed in the next three sections or have him consult the CDC's Web site at http://cdc.gov/nccdphp/dnpa/physical/measuring/index.htm.

TABLE 6.1 **Examples of Activities of Varying Intensity Levels**

Activity type	Moderate	Vigorous
Housework	Vacuuming carpet Cleaning windows Scrubbing floors	Moving furniture Shoveling snow Chopping wood
Occupation	Walking briskly at work	Using heavy tools Fire fighting Loading and unloading a truck Laying bricks
Leisure	Ballroom dancing	Pop dancing
Gardening	Raking Mowing (push mower) Weeding	Shoveling Carrying moderate to heavy loads Tilling Transplanting shrubs
Sports	Volleyball Table tennis Golf without a cart Tai chi Frisbee	Jumping rope Basketball Racquetball Soccer Mountain or rock climbing
Walking	Walking 15-20 minutes/mile	Running Stair climbing

Use the Talk Test

The talk test is one way to help your client understand what you mean by light-, moderate-, and vigorous-intensity activities. A person should be able to sing while doing light activities. When active at a moderate intensity, the person should be able to carry on a conversation comfortably. If a person is too winded or out of breath to carry on a conversation, the activity can be considered vigorous.

Monitor Target Heart Rate

A client can also monitor her heart rate during physical activity to see whether she is within the target zone. For moderate-intensity physical activity, your client should aim for a heart rate that is 60 to 76% of her maximum heart rate, which is based on her age. To estimate a person's maximum age-related heart rate, subtract her age from 220. Then calculate the 60% and 76% levels to obtain the moderate-intensity target range. For example, the estimated maximum age-related heart rate for a 50-year-old woman would be 220 − 50 years = 170 beats per minute (bpm). The target range for moderate-intensity activity would be as follows:

> 60% level: 170 bpm $\times$ 0.60 = 102 bpm
>
> 76% level: 170 bpm $\times$ 0.76 = 129 bpm

You have determined that moderate-intensity physical activity for this 50-year-old woman requires a heart rate that remains between 102 and 129 bpm during physical activity. For vigorous activity, her heart rate should be 77 to 85% of her maximum age-related heart rate. We describe how to take heart rate by palpation a bit later in this chapter in the Tracking the Resting Heart Rate section.

Utilizing Borg's Rating of Perceived Exertion (RPE)

Perceived exertion is based on physical sensations your client may experience during physical activity, including increased heart rate, increased breathing rate, sweating, and muscle fatigue. Although this is a subjective measure, it appears to be a good estimate of actual heart rate (Borg, 1998). It also has the advantage over target heart rate in that it does not require a person to stop his activity to determine how hard he is working (Heyward, 2006). The person can slow down or speed up movement to adjust the intensity of his activity. The Borg scale also is the preferred method to determine intensity for people who are taking medications that affect heart rate or pulse (e.g., beta blockers, calcium channel blockers).

To determine physical activity intensity level, the person simply uses the Borg Rating of Perceived Exertion scale, which ranges from 6 (no exertion) to 20 (maximal exertion). The client is encouraged to focus on his total level of exertion and not one specific aspect, such as leg pain or shortness of breath, and to base his rating on his own feeling of effort rather than on how it might compare to other people's. A rating of 9 (very light) is for low-intensity activities such as taking a slow walk at one's own pace. A rating of 12 to 14 (somewhat hard) suggests that the activity is being performed at moderate intensity, whereas a rating of 15 or higher (hard) is at vigorous intensity.

Tracking Physical Activity Behavior

Lack of time is a primary barrier for many people in their pursuit of a physically active lifestyle. This is why teaching your clients to keep track of how they spend their time is important. Once you understand how a client spends her time, you can work with her to turn time spent in sedentary behavior and light activity into time spent in moderate-intensity physical activity. For example, you can suggest that she replace time spent watching the kids play in the backyard with time spent bike riding or taking a nature walk with the kids. By reorganizing how she spends her time, she does not have to find more time for physical activity.

Have your client keep track of the amount of time she spends in light-, moderate-, and vigorous-intensity activities. She should mark down her activity soon after performing it rather than try to remember everything she did over the course of a week. Figure 6.1 is a form your clients can use to keep track of this information. You can photocopy this form or use it as a starting point for creating your own with the information that you think is important for your clients to record. Using the form in figure 6.1, a client can keep track of 10-minute bouts of activity, 30-minute bouts, or both, whichever you or your client prefers.

We recommend tracking 10-minute bouts of activity at a minimum because this is the minimum duration of activity associated with health benefits (Haskell et al., 2007). Also, because it is an easy number to remember, the accuracy of recording should be fairly good. However, if your client is very sedentary, she might need to start off by tracking 2- or 5-minute bouts until she is able to work up to 10-minute bouts. She can become more active over time by adding 10-minute bouts of activity each day until she accumulates at least 30 minutes each day. If she prefers to accumulate all 30 minutes in one bout of activity, she can report this on the form also.

Even though we don't know the benefits of light activity (e.g., dusting, light stretching, golf using a cart), you may want a client to record time spent in light activity because this information can give you some ideas on how to help him find time in the day to turn some of this light activity into moderate-intensity activity. For example, strolling in the mall window shopping could be stepped up to walking at a moderate pace. If your client is not sure whether the activity was light, moderate, or vigorous, he should consider whether the effort was more like a slow walk at 2 miles (3.2 km) per hour (light activity), a brisk walk at 3 to 4 miles (4.8 to 6.4 km) per hour (moderate activity), or a run (vigorous activity). At the end of each week, you or your client can add up the number of minutes checked for each activity category. You and your

BISHOP BURTON COLLEGE

Activity	Intensity level	10-minute bouts	30-minute bouts	Total minutes
Housework	Light			
	Moderate/ vigorous			
Occupation	Light			
	Moderate/ vigorous			
Leisure	Light			
	Moderate/ vigorous			
Gardening	Light			
	Moderate/ vigorous			
Sports	Light			
	Moderate/ vigorous			
Walking	Light			
	Moderate/ vigorous			
Stairs	Light			
	Moderate/ vigorous			

FIGURE 6.1 Blank activity tracking sheet.

From B. Marcus and L. Forsyth, 2009, *Motivating people to be physically active*, 2nd ed. (Champaign, IL: Human Kinetics).

client can use this information to set realistic goals for improving his level of physical activity, to design a specific activity program, and to determine whether he has met his goals.

Let's look at an example of how to use the activity tracking sheet with a sedentary client. Natalie is a 43-year-old mother of two who works as a sales representative. She was interested in increasing her physical activity level to maintain her weight and improve her energy level. Her activity tracking sheet, presented in figure 6.2, shows that she does a lot of light activity during the week (between work and home) but very little moderate or vigorous activity. Thus, one important strategy for working with Natalie is to determine which of the light activities could be performed at a moderate intensity. She does not appear to have a time barrier because she is already spending time being

Activity	Intensity level	10-minute bouts	30-minute bouts	Total minutes
Housework	Light	*****		50
	Moderate/ vigorous			0
Occupation	Light	*******	****	190
	Moderate/ vigorous			0
Leisure	Light	****		40
	Moderate/ vigorous			0
Gardening	Light	**		20
	Moderate/ vigorous			0
Sports	Light			0
	Moderate/ vigorous			0
Walking	Light	********	*	120
	Moderate/ vigorous	**		20
Stairs	Light	****		40
	Moderate/ vigorous			0

FIGURE 6.2   Filled-out activity tracking sheet.

Reprinted, by permission, from S.N. Blair et al. 2001, *Active living every day* (Champaign, IL: Human Kinetics), 12.

active. Instead, her exercise counselor focused on helping her turn some of her light-intensity activity into moderate-intensity activity. For example, instead of leisurely walking to different parts of the building at work, she stepped up the pace and included taking the stairs instead of the elevator whenever she could. She also stepped up the pace when taking the dog for a walk. She decided to do some of the raking, push mowing, and garden chores instead of leaving these activities for her husband. Finally, she invited some of her friends to go walking with her, rather than talking on the phone with them while she paced around the house. Completing the activity tracking form helped her to see that rather than squeezing in more activity, she could turn light-intensity activities into moderate-intensity ones.

Tracking Time

To help your client find more time to be physically active, you must find out how he spends his work and leisure time. This information can help the two of you find times in the day when he is sedentary and could do some physical activity. Further, it can aid him in finding bouts of activity that can be lengthened—for example, 2-minute bouts of activity that could be turned into 5-minute bouts and 5-minute bouts that could be turned into 10-minute bouts. Only by understanding his activity patterns can you help him to change these patterns. Have your client choose two weekdays and one weekend day in an upcoming week during which to track his activities. Instruct him to carry a worksheet such as the one in figure 6.3 on each of these 3 days and to record exactly what he does with his time. Figure 6.4 is a partial filled-out example.

After your client has recorded his activities, you can determine how many minutes he spends doing any type of physical activity and how many minutes he spends in sedentary pursuits (such as watching television or driving). The more specific your client can be, the more useful this activity will be for you both.

After your client tracks his physical activity habits, it is time to put this information to work to help him become more active. First, look for patterns in the tracking forms that your client has filled out. Does your client tend to be sedentary for the entire workday? If so, a 10-minute walk once each workday might be a great way to help him on his way to a more active lifestyle. Another pattern to look for is time spent in light activity. Help your client to turn strolls into brisk walks, elevator rides into stair climbing, and light yard work into more vigorous yard work. The tracking forms are tools to help you individualize a program to help your client succeed.

Calculating Activity With a Step Counter

Step counters can be an excellent way to quantify amounts of activity. Although many come with extra features such as calculators of distance covered or calories burned, these are unnecessary and often inaccurate. The goal is for

Date: _____ Day of the week: _____

Time slot	Activities, chores, errands, work, child care, leisure	Physically active?	
		Yes	No
7:00 a.m. to 9:00 a.m.			
9:00 a.m. to 11:00 a.m.			
11:00 a.m. to 1:00 p.m.			
1:00 p.m. to 3:00 p.m.			
3:00 p.m. to 5:00 p.m.			
5:00 p.m. to 7:00 p.m.			
7:00 p.m. to 9:00 p.m.			

(continued) ▷

FIGURE 6.3   Time tracking sheet.

From B. Marcus and L. Forsyth, 2009, *Motivating people to be physically active*, 2nd ed. (Champaign, IL: Human Kinetics).

Time slot	Activities, chores, errands, work, child care, leisure	Physically active?	
		Yes	No
9:00 p.m. to 11:00 p.m.			
11:00 p.m. to 1:00 a.m.			
1:00 a.m. to 3:00 a.m.			
3:00 a.m. to 5:00 a.m.			
5:00 a.m. to 7:00 a.m.			

FIGURE 6.3 *(continued)*

From B. Marcus and L. Forsyth, 2009, *Motivating people to be physically active*, 2nd ed. (Champaign, IL: Human Kinetics).

your client to increase her activity. If she gets too hung up on how far she has walked or how many calories she has burned, it may distract her from the goal and thus make meeting it less likely. Also, because distance and calorie calculations are often based on an average person, the values are often inaccurate for the person using them. For example, if your client is short and has a small stride, the readings may be off. Your client is best served with a simple version that just counts steps. (The brand of step counter we prefer and use in our programs is the Yamax Digi-Walker [www.digiwalker.com; pictured on

Date: _____ Day of the week: _____

Time slot	Activities, chores, errands, work, child care, leisure	Physically active?	
		Yes	No
9:00 a.m. to 11:00 a.m.	Work at desk		25 minutes
	Attend meeting		30 minutes
	Walk to friend's desk and back	3 minutes	
	Walk to buy coffee and back	8 minutes	
	Walk to meeting	4 minutes	
	Work at desk		50 minutes
	Total time	**15 minutes**	**105 minutes**
11:00 a.m. to 1:00 p.m.	Walk to local deli and back with friend	10 minutes	
	Eat lunch with friend		20 minutes
	Walk back to desk	5 minutes	
	Work at desk		62 minutes
	Walk to buy coffee and back	8 minutes	
	Coffee break		10 minutes
	Return to office	5 minutes	
	Total time	**28 minutes**	**92 minutes**

FIGURE 6.4 Time tracking example.

Reprinted, by permission, from S.N. Blair et al. 2001, *Active living every day* (Champaign, IL: Human Kinetics), 12.

the next page]. Our studies and those of other researchers have shown this step counter to be the most accurate; it costs from $15 to $25.)

Step counters look a lot like electronic pagers. They contain a small pendulum that moves each time the wearer takes a step. For the greatest accuracy, the wearer must keep the step counter centered over the left hipbone and lined up with the front crease of the slacks. The step counter *must* be firmly attached, so it is best worn on a belt or attached to the waistband of exercise shorts, pants, or undergarments. If your client chooses to wear the step counter on her underwear or pantyhose, she should put it inside, not outside, the waistband. Also, she should be sure to remove the step counter before using the bathroom.

Advise your client to put on the step counter first thing in the morning and keep it on until bedtime. When she takes it off at bedtime, she should record the number of steps she took that day. A sample log sheet is provided

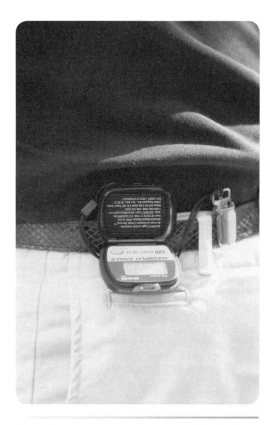

A simple step counter can provide both an assessment of your client's physical activity as well as serve as a source of client feedback toward reaching daily physical activity goals.

in figure 6.5. She should be sure to reset the step counter back to zero for the next day of use.

In studies to date (e.g., Welk et al., 2000), most people accumulate 2,000 to 4,000 steps per day while performing their daily routines (e.g., walking around the house or office, doing daily chores, getting in and out of the car on errands). Walking for 30 minutes at a brisk pace equals about 4,000 steps. These numbers can help you and your client to set realistic short- and long-term goals. Other steps are accumulated through more activity in daily life, such as parking and walking into a fast food restaurant rather than using the drive through and parking at the far end of a shopping mall parking lot. Also, data show that people who are meeting the national guidelines tend to average 10,000 steps or more (Welk et al., 2000).

After your client has recorded her steps for a week, she can calculate her average steps per day. Then you can help her set a reasonable goal and devise a plan for increasing her steps to reach that goal. The long-term goal we usually recommend is 10,000 steps a day, because this has been shown to be

Week: _____

Day of week	Date	Step goal	Actual steps	Minutes of activity	Notes
Sunday					
Monday					
Tuesday					
Wednesday					
Thursday					
Friday					
Saturday					

FIGURE 6.5 **Step counter log.**

From B. Marcus and L. Forsyth, 2009, *Motivating people to be physically active*, 2nd ed. (Champaign, IL: Human Kinetics). Reprinted, by permission, from S.N. Blair et al., 2001, *Active living every day* (Champaign, IL: Human Kinetics), 49.

enough to obtain important health benefits (Welk et al., 2000). However, for a client who is taking only 2,500 steps per day, you may *not* want to talk with her about a long-term goal of obtaining 10,000 steps per day. Rather, you may want to set a goal of 5,000 steps per day, which is more easily attainable for a person at that activity level. Once she has met this goal, the two of you can reevaluate and set the next goal. You may want to create a form for her to use to track her progress over time, such as the example in figure 6.6. A simple graph that you or your client fills out can be a useful way to demonstrate that she has made great progress or has some room to improve.

Step counters can help your clients stay on track. You may want to instruct them to check regularly to see how many steps they have taken. If it's already midafternoon and a client has accumulated only 1,500 steps, he needs to find a way to get in a lot more activity that day. He may need to think creatively about how to get in some purposeful activity, such as taking a 20-minute walk home from the commuter rail station rather than getting a ride with a neighbor or taking a 10-minute walk rather than a coffee break in the afternoon.

Assessing Fitness

We have described means for measuring your clients' time spent engaging in physical activities and patterns of behavior. Understanding these patterns is critical to helping them see more benefits and fewer barriers to living an active lifestyle and to enhancing their motivation to become more physically active. However, actual physical fitness is also an important factor in increasing clients' levels of physical activity. If a client has a very high resting heart rate and cannot walk even half a mile (0.8 km) without becoming breathless,

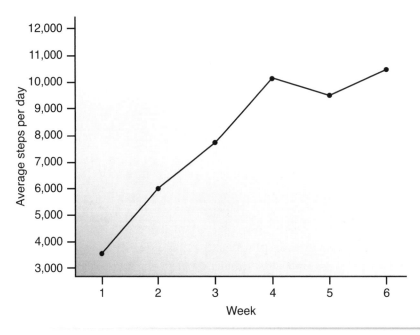

FIGURE 6.6 A weekly goal chart showing the average number of steps taken per day can motivate your client to increase the number of steps she takes per day.

he needs to start an activity program very slowly, even if he is extremely motivated to change. For example, this client could start off performing 2-minute bouts of activity and then slowly move up to 5- and then 10-minute bouts. On the other hand, if your client is fit enough to easily accomplish a half-mile walk but believes she is too busy to be active, your physical activity plan may focus more on rearranging her schedule. You can encourage this client to turn light activity into moderate-intensity activity and to string short bouts of activity together into longer bouts of activity without necessarily adding to her busy day. Activity pattern assessment and physical fitness assessment work hand in hand to help you customize a program that will best meet your client's needs. It is important to develop a plan that she can start and stick with, thereby enhancing the likelihood that she will eventually be active on a daily basis. We will now give you a couple of simple strategies for assessing your client's fitness level. The following two sections give detailed information about assessing a client's physical fitness, physical readiness for more activity, or both (refer to Heyward, 2006 for more in-depth information on physical fitness assessment).

Tracking the Resting Heart Rate

One of the simplest ways to gauge changes in fitness is to track the resting heart rate (beats per minute). As a client's fitness improves, his resting heart

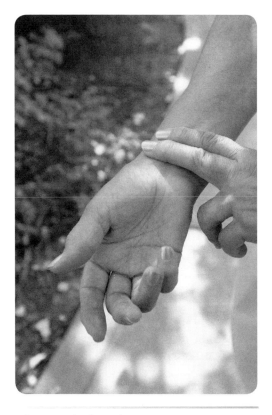

Taking a pulse by palpation.

rate slows down. This happens because when a person increases his fitness level, his heart gets stronger and can pump more blood with each beat, as compared to when he is less fit.

Your clients may not know how to measure their resting heart rate. The easiest place to find a pulse is the inside of the wrist, just below the thumb. Help your client learn how to place his index and middle fingers lightly against the artery at that location. He may need to move his fingers around a bit until he is able to feel the rhythmic beat of his pulse. Next, using a second hand on a watch or a stopwatch, have him count how many times his heart beats in one minute. Then he can record it on a form like the one shown in figure 6.7. Ideally, to ensure the accuracy of this measure, advise your client to record his heart rate first thing in the morning, before getting out of bed, or before he has had any coffee or cigarettes, as either of these stimulants could greatly affect his resting heart rate.

Depending on your situation and your plans for working with your client, you may prefer to measure and record the client's resting heart rate rather than have him do it. If your client has numerous risk factors for heart disease

Date	Resting heart rate	Notes

FIGURE 6.7   **Resting heart rate log.**

From B. Marcus and L. Forsyth, 2009, *Motivating people to be physically active*, 2nd ed. (Champaign, IL: Human Kinetics).

and has repeatedly tried but failed to become more active, you may want to be more proactive. However, if you are working with a more motivated person who wants to work with you only briefly and then work more independently, it is probably best to give him more autonomy from the beginning and teach him how to record his heart rate on his own.

Every month (or whatever interval makes sense in your situation) have your client measure and record his resting heart rate. If he is participating in physical activity regularly, his resting heart rate should decrease over time. Depending on the circumstances, you may also want your client to record whether he is experiencing any extreme emotions such as stress, worry, or sadness. Strong emotional responses can affect heart rate and may help you to interpret unexpected patterns in heart rate over time.

Walking Test

A simple and inexpensive way to assess changes in fitness is a walking test. Your client needs access to a half-mile (0.8 km) track or can map out her own half-mile route. Alternatively, you can suggest a route near the facility where you work with this client. Be sure she warms up first by walking slowly for a few minutes. Then you can time her, or have her time herself, as she walks this route as quickly as possible. In some settings, it may be efficient for a group of people (e.g., employees) to perform this test at the same time. You or your client should record how long it takes to walk the half mile and her heart rate immediately after she finishes. This will help you determine how hard she was working while she walked that distance (figure 6.8). Advise your client to refrain from cigarette smoking and coffee and cola consumption for

Date	Time to walk half mile (minutes and seconds)	Heart rate at end

FIGURE 6.8 Walking test log.

From B. Marcus and L. Forsyth, 2009, *Motivating people to be physically active*, 2nd ed. (Champaign, IL: Human Kinetics). Reprinted, by permission, from S.N. Blair et al., 2001, *Active living every day* (Champaign, IL: Human Kinetics), 120.

at least 1 hour prior to this walking test because these stimulants can raise the heart rate. The client should repeat this test in approximately 3 months to determine her progress.

Assessing Physical Activity and Fitness in Group Settings

All of the methods for measuring physical activity patterns and physical fitness described in this chapter can be used in settings involving more than one client at a time. Instructions for filling out the forms for determining physical activity habits can be given to a group; then people can fill them out individually, and you can provide individual feedback. If the size of the group precludes individual meetings, you may be able to provide feedback to small groups who are confronting similar issues, depending on the confidentiality requirements in your setting.

Another way to use these materials would be to put detailed instructions and forms on a Web site that is password protected (to maintain privacy and confidentiality) and available only to your clients. This allows you to provide individualized feedback and answers to questions via e-mail, a chat room, or an electronic bulletin board.

The physical fitness assessments can also be administered to a group. Similarly, a Web site can be used to provide clients with various half-mile walking routes in their local areas as well as the tracking forms to record and track their changes over time.

Conclusion

In this chapter we explained why it is important to understand and track your clients' physical activity patterns and physical fitness, and we provided you with strategies that will be helpful in accomplishing these objectives. We also provided tools for tracking your clients' activity habits because tracking these habits is critical in helping them to come up with realistic, measurable goals for change. Finally, we described how to use the methods presented in this chapter with more than one client at a time. Now that you are familiar with assessment methods, you are ready to learn about applying the stages of change model in your work with clients.

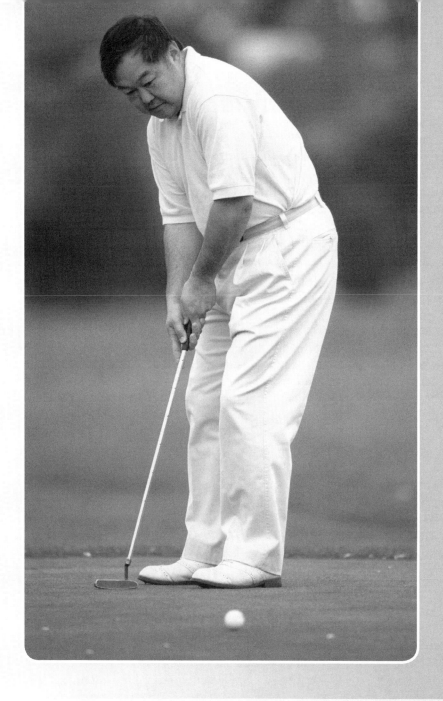

CHAPTER 7

Using the Stages Model in Individual Counseling

The transtheoretical model was originally developed to better understand how people change behavior on their own. The goal was to discover the key ingredients in behavior change so that counselors and therapists could use these ingredients with people who want to change their behaviors but are unwilling to do so on their own. This chapter on applying the stages of change model focuses on individual counseling. The professional can help clients set goals for activity, address problems that arise, and use clients' past histories of behavior change to achieve their current goals.

In this chapter we describe how to assess clients' physical readiness as well as psychological readiness to start a program of physical activity. We explain why it is important to examine clients' past experiences with changing habits and how to help them solve problems that may be getting in the way of becoming more active. We also describe strategies for enhancing clients' confidence that they can change their behavior and for helping them set realistic goals for behavior change. Each of these issues is pertinent at all stages of motivational readiness because of the cyclical nature of behavior change. Therefore, many of the areas described in this chapter need to be addressed repeatedly during the initiation, adoption, and maintenance of physical activity habits. However, these topics are addressed slightly differently for people at each stage. The Stage-Specific Strategies section at the end of this chapter provides some ideas for how you can apply each topic at each stage of motivational readiness when working with individuals. One of the first steps in individual counseling is to assess the client's stage of motivational readiness for physical activity. You should keep this stage in mind as you work with her using the strategies discussed in this chapter.

Physical Readiness

In chapter 1 we described the numerous health benefits of an active lifestyle. Although most people benefit from participating in programs of regular physical activity, those with health problems may need more medical supervision than you or your facility can provide. Thus, it is important to first assess your client's physical readiness for physical activity before embarking on specific physical activity counseling.

Depending on your professional training, you may or may not feel comfortable addressing the issue of safety with your client. In general, exercising at a moderate intensity (as opposed to vigorously) is safe for most people. For most people, a medical exam or stress test is not required before increasing moderate-intensity physical activities. Nevertheless, people with diseases such as heart disease and diabetes should check with their doctors before beginning to exercise even at a moderate intensity. One often-used method of determining whether a person can safely increase activity is the Physical Activity Readiness Questionnaire (PAR-Q; figure 7.1). Your client should read the questionnaire carefully and answer each yes-or-no question honestly.

Physical Activity Readiness
Questionnaire - PAR-Q
(revised 2002)

PAR-Q & YOU

(A Questionnaire for People Aged 15 to 69)

Regular physical activity is fun and healthy, and increasingly more people are starting to become more active every day. Being more active is very safe for most people. However, some people should check with their doctor before they start becoming much more physically active.

If you are planning to become much more physically active than you are now, start by answering the seven questions in the box below. If you are between the ages of 15 and 69, the PAR-Q will tell you if you should check with your doctor before you start. If you are over 69 years of age, and you are not used to being very active, check with your doctor.

Common sense is your best guide when you answer these questions. Please read the questions carefully and answer each one honestly: check YES or NO.

YES	NO		
☐	☐	1.	Has your doctor ever said that you have a heart condition __and__ that you should only do physical activity recommended by a doctor?
☐	☐	2.	Do you feel pain in your chest when you do physical activity?
☐	☐	3.	In the past month, have you had chest pain when you were not doing physical activity?
☐	☐	4.	Do you lose your balance because of dizziness or do you ever lose consciousness?
☐	☐	5.	Do you have a bone or joint problem (for example, back, knee or hip) that could be made worse by a change in your physical activity?
☐	☐	6.	Is your doctor currently prescribing drugs (for example, water pills) for your blood pressure or heart condition?
☐	☐	7.	Do you know of __any other reason__ why you should not do physical activity?

If **you** **answered**

YES to one or more questions

Talk with your doctor by phone or in person BEFORE you start becoming much more physically active or BEFORE you have a fitness appraisal. Tell your doctor about the PAR-Q and which questions you answered YES.

• You may be able to do any activity you want — as long as you start slowly and build up gradually. Or, you may need to restrict your activities to those which are safe for you. Talk with your doctor about the kinds of activities you wish to participate in and follow his/her advice.

• Find out which community programs are safe and helpful for you.

NO to all questions

If you answered NO honestly to __all__ PAR-Q questions, you can be reasonably sure that you can:

• start becoming much more physically active – begin slowly and build up gradually. This is the safest and easiest way to go.

• take part in a fitness appraisal – this is an excellent way to determine your basic fitness so that you can plan the best way for you to live actively. It is also highly recommended that you have your blood pressure evaluated. If your reading is over 144/94, talk with your doctor before you start becoming much more physically active.

DELAY BECOMING MUCH MORE ACTIVE:

• if you are not feeling well because of a temporary illness such as a cold or a fever – wait until you feel better; or

• if you are or may be pregnant – talk to your doctor before you start becoming more active.

PLEASE NOTE: If your health changes so that you then answer YES to any of the above questions, tell your fitness or health professional. Ask whether you should change your physical activity plan.

Informed Use of the PAR-Q: The Canadian Society for Exercise Physiology, Health Canada, and their agents assume no liability for persons who undertake physical activity, and if in doubt after completing this questionnaire, consult your doctor prior to physical activity.

No changes permitted. You are encouraged to photocopy the PAR-Q but only if you use the entire form.

NOTE: If the PAR-Q is being given to a person before he or she participates in a physical activity program or a fitness appraisal, this section may be used for legal or administrative purposes.

"I have read, understood and completed this questionnaire. Any questions I had were answered to my full satisfaction."

NAME _____

SIGNATURE _____ DATE _____

SIGNATURE OF PARENT _____ WITNESS _____
or GUARDIAN (for participants under the age of majority)

Note: This physical activity clearance is valid for a maximum of 12 months from the date it is completed and becomes invalid if your condition changes so that you would answer YES to any of the seven questions.

CSEP
SCPE © Canadian Society for Exercise Physiology

Supported by: ▮◆▮ Health Santé
Canada Canada

continued on other side...

FIGURE 7.1 **Page one of the Physical Activity Readiness Questionnaire.**

From *Physical Activity Readiness Questionnaire* (PAR-Q) © 2002. Used with permission from the Canadian Society for Exercise Physiology. http://www.csep.ca.

Clients who answer yes to one or more questions on the PAR-Q should speak with their doctors before increasing their physical activity. They should be sure to tell their doctors the specific questions to which they answered yes.

Clients who answer no to all the questions can begin activity slowly and increase it gradually; it is your job to tell them how to do this. If you work with clients for more than 6 months, periodically readminister the PAR-Q and have any clients who answer yes to any of the questions contact their doctors.

People who come to you for help are likely to be sedentary; therefore, they should begin with moderate-intensity activities. However, if they want to exercise vigorously, they should check with a doctor first if one of the following applies:

- Is a man 45 or older or a woman 55 or older
- Has *two* or more of the following risk factors: has a family history of heart disease, is a current cigarette smoker, has high blood pressure, has high cholesterol, has high blood sugar, is 30 pounds (13.6 kg) overweight or more, or is currently not at all active
- Has heart or blood vessel disease, diabetes, lung disease, asthma, thyroid disorder, or kidney disease

Physical Activity History

Once you have determined that clients can safely increase their physical activity, it is helpful to learn more about their past experiences with physical activity. Questionnaire 7.1 in appendix A will help you determine how long it has been since they were more physically active, some of the reasons they stopped being physically active in the past, and the types of activities they may have previously enjoyed. The information from this questionnaire can be useful as you plan individual or group programs. For clients who are currently inactive or underactive, we encourage you to look for patterns in their responses in this questionnaire so that you can prevent similar relapses from occurring this time around. You also may want to readminister this questionnaire as necessary to be aware of clients' shifting priorities.

Psychological Readiness

Psychological readiness, not physical readiness, is likely to be the main barrier to activity for most of your clients. Although you might not see a lot of stage 1 people in the setting in which you work, chances are good that you see lots of stage 2 clients—people who keep meaning to start some physical activity but never get around to it. You may also see people in stage 3, who do some physical activity but have not quite figured out how to make it a habit of sufficient frequency and duration to obtain important health benefits. Your task with all your clients is to aid them in moving through the stages of change and help them avoid pitfalls on what can be an arduous journey. You must help them understand how their behavior regarding physical activity is like other behaviors they have succeeded in changing in the past. You should help them examine the benefits of and barriers to changing their behavior and assist them in solving problems that arise when they try to change their physical activity habits. You also need to aid them in building confidence in themselves and in setting realistic goals that they can achieve to make them feel proud and successful.

Personal Successes and Past Behavior Change

Some clients may want to be more active but tell you that they do not believe they can succeed. They are overwhelmed by the idea of changing their whole lives to become more active. One very effective tool for working with clients like these is to sidestep the issue of physical activity initially. Instead, start off by helping them to recall some other lifestyle change they made, with or without professional help. This is key because past behavior is the single strongest predictor of future behavior. Helping clients recall past successes is likely to empower them to make positive changes in their physical activity habits.

Have your client take a few minutes to relate one or more success stories: a healthy habit she has adopted or an unhealthy habit she has stopped. Then ask her to think about why she was able to make the change. What helped her succeed? What got in her way? For example, if she quit smoking by setting her 40th birthday as her quit date and receiving support from family, friends, and coworkers, this gives you both a lot of information that might help her start a program of regular physical activity. Figure 7.2 is an example of a form you and your client might use to record these successes.

Once you and your client have discussed past successes and how she achieved them, you should have a lot of useful information about the strategies that work and do not work for her. This information can help you to work with her areas of strength (e.g., a lot of supportive friends) and deal with areas of weakness or difficulty (e.g., a very stressful work environment). In this way you can create a program that is uniquely suited to her and thus extremely likely to help her achieve her goals.

Let's say you learn that when your client took a Thursday and Friday off from work and spent Thursday, Friday, Saturday, and Sunday surrounded by supportive friends and away from her stressful job, she was able to radically decrease the amount of coffee she consumed. This was a personal goal because her primary care physician had told her that decreased caffeine consumption might help decrease the frequency and intensity of her headaches. By the time your client returned to work the next Monday, she had established a new habit of making every other cup of coffee decaffeinated. She was able to maintain this new habit with phone calls and e-mail from supportive friends over the next two weeks. This information about your client's past provides

---

Habits I've changed

    1. _____

    2. _____

    3. _____

Things that helped me succeed

    1. _____

    2. _____

    3. _____

Obstacles that got in my way

    1. _____

    2. _____

    3. _____

FIGURE 7.2   Record of past successes.

From B. Marcus and L. Forsyth, 2009, *Motivating people to be physically active*, 2nd ed. (Champaign, IL: Human Kinetics).

many important clues for helping her change her physical activity behavior. Where are those friends now? How can she mobilize them? Can she take a couple of days off from work, or can she take 60 rather than 30 minutes for lunch so that she can fit in some physical activity?

Readiness to Change Physical Activity Habits

Some people believe that we just need to make up our minds to do something and then we can do it, relying on a lot of willpower in the process. However, most behavior change happens slowly, and lasting behavior change occurs only when a person is motivated to change. Although some people can make major lifestyle changes on their own, many need help, often from professionals like you.

How does a client know that he is ready to change a behavior? One way is to ask himself, *What will I get as a result of making this behavior change? (i.e., what are the benefits of change?)*. If he cannot come up with at least a few key benefits, he is unlikely to accomplish even short-term change at this point. Have him take a few moments to write down his reasons for wanting to change his activity habits. This exercise is useful for clients at all stages of motivational readiness (even stage 1 people can list lots of reasons to become more active, they just have not acted on them) because understanding the benefits of exercise is critical for adopting and sticking with a physically active lifestyle.

Another important component to changing behavior is determining what your client will have to give up or what he will find unpleasant if he makes a change. It is unrealistic to think that a person can make a major life transition such as becoming regularly active from being primarily inactive without having some aspects of the process be annoying or frustrating. Barriers to behavior change might get in the way of your client's best-laid plans. For example, if your client is worried that his family will feel burdened or neglected as a result of his physical activity, you should discuss this with him. Have him take a few minutes to generate a list of any barriers to physical activity behavior change. Sample forms for listing both benefits of and barriers to physical activity are presented in figures 7.3 and 7.4.

With your client, look over his list of barriers to physical activity and examine the number and nature of the barriers. Help him determine which are true barriers and which are excuses. For example, an unsafe neighborhood is a legitimate barrier to walking in the dark after work. However, preferring to spend leisure time window-shopping rather than being active is just an excuse to not exercise. Work on problem-solving exercises to determine which are true barriers. Once you have identified the true barriers, you are in a position to address them. You can teach your client how to find time in his day to be physically active. You can guide him in turning light activity into moderate-intensity activity. However, he may well come up with more excuses, which can put you in a cyclical conversation that leaves you both frustrated. One strategy for problem solving is described in the next section.

Benefits of physical activity

1. _____

2. _____

3. _____

4. _____

5. _____

6. _____

7. _____

8. _____

FIGURE 7.3 Record of benefits of physical activity.

From B. Marcus and L. Forsyth, 2009, *Motivating people to be physically active*, 2nd ed. (Champaign, IL: Human Kinetics).

Barriers to physical activity

1. _____
2. _____
3. _____
4. _____
5. _____
6. _____
7. _____
8. _____

FIGURE 7.4 Record of barriers to physical activity.

From B. Marcus and L. Forsyth, 2009, *Motivating people to be physically active*, 2nd ed. (Champaign, IL: Human Kinetics).

The IDEA Approach to Problem Solving

Once your client has identified her barriers to being physically active, the next step is to help her use some simple problem-solving skills. Problem solving means thinking creatively about the most effective solution to use when a problem gets in the way. Thinking creatively is key. Encourage your client to be as creative as possible when coming up with solutions. Sometimes the most absurd solution actually works best! Once she has come up with a variety of possible solutions, help her choose one to try out first; you can determine later how well it worked. She should pick a good time to implement her solutions to enhance the likelihood of success. Emphasize that finding out that one solution does not work is not bad news. This information can help you both find a better solution that not only works but also can be maintained over time. The concept of looking for alternative solutions when one does not pan out helps to counter all-or-nothing thinking, which often keeps a person from making change (e.g., *I can't find the hour necessary to go to the gym right now so I'll wait until work slows down this summer*).

The IDEA technique is a simple problem-solving approach that has worked well in a number of our studies and with a number of our clients. The acronym stands for *identify* the problem, *develop* a list of solutions, *evaluate* the solutions, and *analyze* how well the plan worked. It is easy to implement and can be helpful to all clients, especially those who cannot see past their barriers to behavior change. The goal is to help clients discover new options, move out of their current situations, and emerge into the new situations they say they want yet have been unable to create.

Identify the Problem   The first step of the IDEA approach is to have your client select one barrier and write it down on the IDEA form in figure 7.5 found at the end of this chapter. Ask your client to think about how this barrier specifically keeps her from being active. Next, ask her to write down the most important details about this personal barrier. For example, if her barrier is frequent business travel, she may say that she is concerned specifically about her personal safety when she is away from home.

Develop a List of Solutions   Help your client brainstorm and come up with as many creative solutions as possible. If she has trouble thinking up solutions, step in and offer some. Be sure to think broadly and to keep in mind what your client has already revealed about herself. That is, try to personalize your responses as much as possible. Encourage her not to worry

Identify a barrier that keeps you from being active (or more active, or as active as you would like to be).

_____

_____

_____

Develop a few creative solutions.

_____

_____

_____

Evaluate your list of solutions. In the following space, write the solution you are willing to try and exactly _when_ you will put it into action.

_____

_____

_____

Analyze how well your plan worked and revise it if necessary. If your plan worked well, great! If your plan did not work too well, look back at your list of solutions and try again.

_____

_____

_____

FIGURE 7.5   **IDEA form.**

From B. Marcus and L. Forsyth, 2009, _Motivating people to be physically active_, 2nd ed. (Champaign, IL: Human Kinetics). Adapted, by permission, from S.N. Blair et al., 2001, _Active living every day_ (Champaign, IL: Human Kinetics), 31.

about whether any given solution is good or bad, workable or unrealistic. That can come later. Sometimes a client's seemingly far-fetched idea turns out to be the best solution. Have your client write down all the ideas that come up, and encourage her to keep the list with her for a few days so she can add more solutions as she thinks of them.

Evaluate the Solutions   Some solutions seem more realistic than others. However, solutions that seem far-fetched at first may appear more realistic with more thought. Work with your client to select one solution she is willing to try. Then help her to plan how and when to put it into action. For example, if your client's main barrier is business travel and the specific problem is that she does not feel safe walking in unfamiliar areas, one solution could be to check ahead to make sure the hotel has an exercise facility. If it does not, she can switch hotels, if possible, to one that does have such a facility. Another plan might involve teaching her a set of simple aerobic exercises or a jump rope routine that she can take on the road and do in the safety of her hotel room. A third plan might be to have her walk as much as she can while at the airport and in other heavily traveled areas where she feels safe.

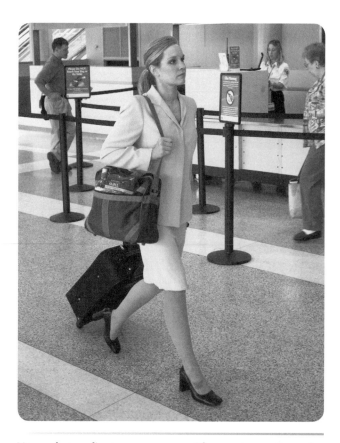

You and your client can come up with some innovative solutions to physical activity barriers using the IDEA approach such as finding a way to power walk during a business trip.

Analyze How Well the Plan Worked   After your client has given her plan a try, help her to analyze how well it worked. Help her to honestly examine what did and did not work. Then help her to revise her plan before she tries it again. For example, if your client planned to rely on a hotel exercise facility but did not get around to calling ahead of time and then found that the hotel did not have a facility, it is clear that her plan did not work because she did not implement it. Thus, there is no reason to throw this plan away; rather, she should try it again. However, if she called ahead to discover that there was an exercise facility, yet it was so crowded from 6 to 8 a.m. that she couldn't exercise before her hectic 9 a.m. to 10 p.m. workday started, it might be necessary to revise the plan and perhaps try the jump rope routine the next time. Because most clients have more than one barrier to address, you can encourage them to use the IDEA form for other barriers once they have used it successfully.

Confidence

Having confidence in oneself is critical during all phases of behavior change. Research in the field of psychology has demonstrated that helping people believe in themselves and visualize themselves as people who are, or one day will be, successful is paramount to helping them think about change, make change, and sustain change over the years. Your job is really twofold. First, you need to regularly convey your belief that your client can and will succeed in his efforts to start or stick with a physical activity plan. Second, you need to teach your client the skills to believe in himself, because this is critical once his contact with you has concluded.

To gauge your client's level of confidence, ask him to rate his confidence that he can start being or continue to be regularly physically active on a scale of 1 to 5, with the lowest level of confidence being 1 and the highest level being 5. (For a more detailed questionnaire to measure confidence, see questionnaire 4.2 in appendix A.)

If your client answers 1 or 2, help him think about why he does not feel confident, and discuss ways to help him become more confident. Pinpointing specific obstacles is often the first step to overcoming them. For example, if your client lacks confidence that he can exercise after work because of family responsibilities, you can suggest that he walk during breaks and lunchtime and thus have already accumulated 30 minutes of physical activity before he goes home.

If your client rates his confidence a 3, he is halfway there. Help him to think about what he likes most and least about physical activity. Do what you can to help make physical activity more enjoyable, convenient, or safe for him. For example, ask whether he prefers to be active alone or with others and whether he prefers to be active during the workday or before or after work. Try to find out why he has these preferences. Perhaps he prefers walking alone because he is embarrassed that he is too unfit to jog, the activity in which many of his friends participate. This may be important information if you learn that your client actually prefers being active with others and aspires to join his friends eventually for early morning jogs.

If your client answered 4 or 5, he is well on his way to making exercise a lifelong habit. Maintaining a physically active lifestyle is extremely challenging. Staying active requires continued time, energy, and planning for a lifetime. To stay regularly active, a person needs to set the alarm clock to go off early in the morning or skip part of lunch to take a walk or stop at the gym on the way home from work every day. Participating in physical activity never ceases to be an issue. Your client may well begin to truly enjoy activity and even look forward to it. However, it always takes thought, time, and planning. Thus, it is critical that he remain confident that he can stick with physical activity even during times of stress, sadness, or extreme pressure at work. Work with him to instill the confidence that he can start up his physical activity program anew if his efforts get derailed for some reason, such as following the birth of his first child or relocation to a new city.

Set Short- and Long-Term Goals

Helping your client determine both short- and long-term goals will help with her activity plan. The goals you set together become the contract you two agree to pursue. For example, if your client's goal is weight loss, her short-term goal may be to walk for 15 minutes daily, her medium-term goal may be to walk for 30 minutes daily, and her long-term goal may be to walk for 60 minutes daily. Your role is to help her achieve those goals. To that end, the clearer her goals are, the better her chances of reaching them will be. Teaching your client effective ways of setting goals can go a long way toward helping her succeed. Figure 7.6 is an example of a form you and your client can use to record goals. Here are three important tips for goal setting:

■ **Be specific.** People who set specific goals do better than people who say, "I'll try to do my best." For example, if your client says, "This week I'll try to be more active," help him to turn this into a specific goal such as, "This week I'll walk for 15 minutes every lunch hour and another 15 minutes after dinner." Specific goals tend to be effective because they are measurable. Goals should also be attainable; with your assistance, your client can set specific goals that she can realistically attain. Goal setting is related to confidence building; if your client reaches a goal he has set, he will have increased confidence that he can progress to meet his next goal.

■ **Set both short-term and long-term goals.** If your client's long-term goal is to walk 1 hour a day, 5 days a week, he should not expect to reach that goal immediately. Help him recognize the need to start off slowly yet never to lose sight of the goal. A good short-term goal might be to walk for three 10-minute bouts each on Sunday, Wednesday, and Friday, then gradually increase the number of minutes and the number of days a week that he

My short-term goal that I plan to achieve next week:

_____

_____

How I plan to monitor my progress on reaching this goal:

_____

_____

My long-term goal I plan to achieve by _____(date):

_____

_____

How I plan to monitor my progress on reaching this goal:

_____

_____

FIGURE 7.6   **Goal-setting form.**

From B. Marcus and L. Forsyth, 2009, *Motivating people to be physically active,* 2nd ed. (Champaign, IL: Human Kinetics). Adapted, by permission, from S.N. Blair et al., 2001, *Active living every day* (Champaign, IL: Human Kinetics), 31.

walks. In this way, he builds confidence that he can meet the goals he sets, which will then empower him to set future goals. Reaching one's goal creates a sense of mastery and a warm sense of achievement. Nothing is more important than helping your client attain his long-term goals and then maintain the behaviors that got him there.

■ **Give your client feedback, and teach him to give himself feedback.** Choose a way to track your client's progress. Assessment tools are suggested in chapters 2, 4, and 6. Monitoring progress lets your client see the pattern of ups and downs and helps him understand that the downs are only temporary. He can then learn strategies to turn these downs into ups and to avoid some of these downs in the future.

Measure Success

There are several ways to measure success in physical activity. You can help your client add up the time she spends doing an activity and set a goal for increasing her activity time. You can also use any of the questionnaires in appendix A, readministering them every 3 months to evaluate your client's progress. You and your client can also evaluate the new strategies she has learned and other strategies that may be helpful in her movement toward becoming more physically active.

Goal setting is valuable only when you can measure success in attaining goals. For your client to feel successful, you and she must agree on what constitutes success. At different points, you may measure success by different means. Initially, success may be measured more by changes in the mediators of change in physical activity described in chapter 4. Later, success may be measured by forward progression in the stages of change as described in chapter 2 or by changes in fitness as described in chapter 6. Measuring success is important for keeping your client on track and ensuring that short- and long-term goals stay realistic.

The following case example illustrates how to use the information presented in this chapter to help a client become more active. As this case shows, the process of becoming more active is not always a smooth one; it often requires repeated problem solving and patience.

CASE EXAMPLE

Creating Change Through Individual Counseling

Rosemary, a 28-year-old single mother, was referred for physical activity counseling by her primary care physician. She had a lifelong history of obesity and knew that managing her weight and lowering her blood pressure would require that she make some changes. She agreed to seek help from a physical activity counselor.

When Rosemary first met with her counselor, she was asked to complete a physical activity history questionnaire (see questionnaire 7.1) and the physical activity stages of change questionnaire (see questionnaire 2.1). From her responses on these assessments, her counselor learned that she had never been physically active for any significant amount of time, but she was in stage 2 (thinking about change). Other measures indicated that she had low self-efficacy for physical activity, identified several barriers that prevented her from being physically active (e.g., low energy, little time, physical discomfort, difficulty finding enjoyable activities), and had made few steps toward becoming more active to date (i.e., scored low on the processes of change questionnaire).

To boost her motivation, Rosemary's counselor discussed what she had to gain by becoming more active, such as weight loss, improved health, increased energy, and becoming a healthy role model for her 4-year-old son. To build her confidence, Rosemary's counselor asked her about other behavior changes she had been able to achieve in the past. Rosemary had struggled with eating healthier, losing weight, and saving money her whole life and felt a bit overwhelmed by trying to incorporate a regular physical activity routine into her life. However, she and her counselor soon identified Rosemary's ability to drink more water rather than soda as a behavior change she had accomplished in the recent past. She did so by setting small goals (drinking one or two glasses of water with meals, then sipping on water while at her workstation), making environmental changes (keeping a water bottle handy and keeping no soda in her house), and creating reminders (placing sticky notes on her refrigerator and on her computer at work). Rosemary and her counselor proceeded to work out a plan for using similar strategies for physical activity. They set a modest weekly goal of three 15-minute walks around the block, and Rosemary was to keep her walking shoes by the door as a reminder. She was concerned about child care, but using the IDEA approach, she and her counselor came up with the solution of having her son ride his bicycle beside her while she walked. Rosemary was excited and left the counselor's office thinking she could do this.

However, at her two-week follow-up appointment, Rosemary admitted that she had procrastinated the first week, and an unexpected spring snowstorm interfered with her goal of walking outside during the week of her appointment. She and her counselor used the IDEA approach to brainstorm about how to be active in her home should the weather be bad. Rosemary mentioned that her mother had an old treadmill in the basement and would most likely be willing to loan it to her. Rosemary agreed to ask to borrow the treadmill, and they kept the goal of three 15-minute walks a week.

The following session, Rosemary again admitted that she had not met her physical activity goal. She kept meaning to clean up the clutter in the living room before she retrieved the treadmill from her mother's house, but she just never got around to it. At this point her counselor was quite concerned that Rosemary was going to become discouraged before she even got started. They briefly reviewed what Rosemary had to gain by increasing her physical activity. Her counselor suggested that it might be worthwhile to increase Rosemary's activity during the workday so that she would be done with her activity goal before she got home and needed to take care of her son and the house.

Although her workplace had an exercise facility available to employees, Rosemary felt too self-conscious about her size to exercise in such a public place. She also was resistant to using her lunch break for taking a walk as that was when she ran errands that she didn't think she would otherwise get done. However, when her counselor suggested that a good way to start might be to use the stairs to get to her third-floor office rather than the elevator three times during the course of a workday, Rosemary perked up. This would not take too much time, would be a way to get in some activity out of view of others, and would be a step in the right direction.

The next time Rosemary met with her counselor, she had good news to report. She had met her goal of using the stairs three times daily and felt encouraged enough to try doing this at the doctor's office and at the mall. Although she was still far from the 60 minutes of daily moderate-intensity activity that was her ultimate goal, this success helped move her to stage 3 (doing some physical activity) and boosted her self-efficacy. Over the course of the next 6 months, she was able to incorporate other activities such as a weekly game of tag with her son, gardening on the weekends, and taking a walk outdoors at least once a week. She and her counselor generated rewards Rosemary could give herself for her progress (e.g., renting favorite movies, taking an afternoon nap on the weekends). She was well on her way to developing a physically active lifestyle.

Stage-Specific Strategies for Individual Counseling

This section provides strategies to use in individual counseling with clients. They are broken down into stages of readiness for change.

STAGE 1

NOT THINKING ABOUT CHANGE

Even though your client is not considering becoming physically active right now, you can still do some brief counseling to help her move toward thinking about behavior change. Here are some ways you can apply the strategies discussed in this chapter for a client in this earliest stage.

Is your client physically ready to begin physical activity?

■ Give your client the PAR-Q (figure 7.1) to identify any health reasons that would preclude physical activity.

■ Explain to your client that moderate-intensity activity is unlikely to cause adverse health events.

■ Refer your client to a physician if any health problems exist.

How has your client successfully changed behavior in the past?

■ Increase your client's confidence by discussing any past attempts at behavior change and identifying strategies that worked then and could help with physical activity change in the future (figure 7.2).

■ Address any problems that have gotten in your client's way during past attempts at behavior change (figure 7.5).

How might your client benefit from physical activity?

■ Ask your client to write down how she might benefit from some physical activity (figure 7.3).

■ Suggest some benefits your client may not have thought of yet.

■ Encourage your client to learn more about the benefits of physical activity.

■ Have your client assess how important these benefits are to her.

What might your client need to give up to become physically active, and what barriers does your client need to address?

■ Ask your client to write down what she would have to give up to become physically active and what she might find unpleasant about physical activity (figure 7.4).

■ Have your client assess how important these issues are to her.

■ Help your client differentiate between true barriers and excuses.

■ Help your client find solutions to these barriers using the IDEA approach (figure 7.5).

STAGE 1

How can you help your client to become more confident about physical activity?

- Let your client know that you believe in her ability to become a physically active person someday.

- Reinforce any action your client takes that can help her think about trying some physical activity (e.g., talking to others about physical activity, reading about it, thinking about how she might benefit if she were to become physically active).

- Ask your client to assess her confidence in someday becoming more active on a scale from 1 (not confident) to 5 (very confident).

- Work on increasing your client's confidence by trying to pinpoint perceived obstacles and developing realistic strategies for overcoming them (figures 7.4 and 7.5).

- Relate your client's past successes at behavior change with her ability to become physically active in the future (figure 7.2).

- Discuss what went wrong during past attempts at behavior change and reframe them as learning experiences that can teach your client what to do differently should she decide to become physically active.

What goals might help your client move toward behavior change?

- Work with your client to set a manageable, short-term goal, perhaps around a mediator of behavior change (see chapter 4) that can help her start thinking about changing her sedentary lifestyle (figure 7.6).

- Ask your client to discuss with her physician how she might personally benefit from some physical activity (comprehending benefits) (figure 7.5).

- Another short-term goal might be to have your client use the IDEA approach on her own to work out a possible solution to one or two of her perceived barriers (decisional balance).

- Ask your client to try to spot a person similar to herself in age, body shape, and health status who is being physically active (self-efficacy).

- Have your client ask a friend or family member to take over child care or household responsibilities for an hour so that she can spend some time reading about physical activity or touring a local facility (enlisting social support; increasing knowledge).

- Ask your client to write down some ways that her sedentary lifestyle is affecting people important to her (caring about consequences to others).

- Agree on something your client can do or a small gift she can buy to reward herself for achieving her goals (rewarding oneself).

- Suggest that your client allow herself to engage in a pleasurable sedentary activity (e.g., watching a favorite movie, surfing the Web, taking a short nap) only after she has accomplished one of her activity-related goals.

(continued) ▷

BISHOP BURTON COLLEGE

STAGE 1

STAGE 1 *(continued)*

- Set up a point system that your client can use to earn a larger reward (e.g., accomplishing a small goal earns 2 points; 20 accumulated points can be used to purchase a night at the movies or some personal time).
- Reinforce the idea that achieving other behavioral or cognitive goals, even if they do not include actual physical activity, are productive and worthwhile.

How can you measure your client's success?

- Reassess your client's stage of change (see chapter 2).
- Consider giving your client the processes of change questionnaire (questionnaire 4.1 in appendix A) to see whether she is using more strategies.
- Measure your client's confidence to see whether it has improved by using the self-efficacy questionnaire (questionnaire 4.2 in appendix A).
- Reassess your client's perceived benefits relative to her perceived barriers using the decisional balance questionnaire (questionnaire 4.4 in appendix A).
- Ask your client to simply rate how satisfied she is with her progress on a scale of 1 to 5.

STAGE 2

THINKING ABOUT CHANGE

Your client is thinking about becoming more active, so your task is to help him commit to a start date and do some planning that will enhance the likelihood that he will be successful in this endeavor and find his physical activity experience pleasant enough to try it again. Here are some ideas for helping a client who is thinking about change but has not yet engaged in any actual physical activity.

Is your client physically ready to begin physical activity?

- Give your client the PAR-Q (figure 7.1) to identify any health reasons that would preclude physical activity.
- Explain to your client that moderate-intensity activity is unlikely to cause adverse health events.
- Refer your client to a physician if any health problems exist or if your client expresses interest in starting with vigorous activity.

How has your client successfully changed behavior in the past?

- Increase your client's self-efficacy by discussing his past attempts at behavior change and identifying strategies that worked then and could help with beginning physical activity (figure 7.2).
- Address any problems that have gotten in the way during past attempts at behavior change and may become an issue for changing physical activity habits (figure 7.5).

How might your client benefit from physical activity?

- Ask your client to write down how he might benefit from physical activity (figure 7.3).
- Suggest some benefits your client may not have thought of yet.
- Encourage your client to learn more about the benefits of physical activity.
- Have your client assess how important these benefits are to him.

What might your client need to give up to become physically active, and what barriers does your client need to address?

- Ask your client to write down what he would have to give up to become physically active and what he might find unpleasant about physical activity (figure 7.4).
- Have your client assess how important these issues are to him.
- Help your client differentiate between true barriers and excuses.
- Help your client find solutions to these barriers using the IDEA approach (figure 7.5).

(continued) ▶

STAGE 2

How can you help your client to become more confident about physical activity?

■ Let your client know that you believe in his ability to become a physically active person.

■ Emphasize that your client has already made progress because he is thinking about becoming physically active.

■ Work on increasing your client's confidence by trying to pinpoint perceived obstacles and developing realistic strategies for overcoming them (figures 7.4 and 7.5).

■ Relate your client's past successes at behavior change with his ability to become physically active in the future (figure 7.2).

■ Discuss what went wrong during past attempts at behavior change and reframe them as learning experiences that can teach your client what to do differently should he decide to become physically active.

■ Begin to identify types of activities that might be manageable and also enjoyable for your client to try when he is ready. Plan when, where, and with whom your client might do these activities so that he can clearly visualize them.

What goals might help your client move toward behavior change?

■ Work with your client to set manageable short- and long-term goals, perhaps around a mediator of behavior change (see chapter 4) that can help him move closer to actually trying some physical activity (figure 7.6).

■ Recommend that your client make a few calls to learn where he might perform his chosen activity (increasing knowledge).

■ Ask your client to try the IDEA approach (figure 7.5) on his own to work out solutions to one or two of the obstacles that seem to get in the way of actually trying some activity (decisional balance).

■ Recommend that your client ask someone close to him to help solve some of the problems that are holding him back (enlisting social support).

■ Suggest that your client commit himself to actually trying a brief, manageable bout of physical activity, such as a 5-minute walk (self-efficacy; committing oneself).

■ Ask your client to look up how many calories are burned for some of the activities he thinks he would be likely to do (outcome expectations).

■ Ask your client to complete a personal time study like that found in chapter 6 (e.g., monitoring time spent in sedentary pursuits and in physical activity for a typical weekday and weekend day; increasing knowledge).

■ Ask your client to write down some ways his sedentary lifestyle is affecting people important to him (caring about consequences to others).

- Agree on something your client can do or a small gift he can buy to reward himself for achieving his goals (rewarding oneself).

- Suggest that your client allow himself to engage in a pleasurable sedentary activity (e.g., watching a favorite movie, surfing the Web, taking a short nap) only after he has accomplished one of his activity goals.

- Set up a point system that your client can use to earn a larger reward (e.g., accomplishing a small goal earns 2 points; 20 accumulated points can be used to purchase a weekend at a bed and breakfast).

- Reinforce the idea that achieving goals, even if they do not include actual physical activity, is productive and worthwhile.

Has your client been successful in moving toward becoming physically active?

- Reassess your client's stage of change (see chapter 2).

- Consider giving your client the processes of change questionnaire (questionnaire 4.1 in appendix A).

- Measure your client's confidence by using the self-efficacy questionnaire (questionnaire 4.2 in appendix A) to see whether it has improved.

- Reassess your client's perceived benefits relative to his perceived barriers using the decisional balance questionnaire (questionnaire 4.4 in appendix A).

- Ask your client to simply rate how satisfied he is with his progress on a scale of 1 to 5.

STAGE 3

DOING SOME PHYSICAL ACTIVITY

Your client is doing some physical activity but not enough, so you need to help her develop some additional strategies for increasing her activity level. Here are some ideas for a client in this stage.

Is your client physically ready to increase physical activity?

- Give your client the PAR-Q (figure 7.1) to identify any health reasons that would preclude physical activity.
- Explain to your client that moderate-intensity activity is unlikely to cause adverse health events.
- Refer your client to a physician if any health problems exist or if your client expresses interest in starting to do vigorous-intensity activity and has one of the risk factors mentioned earlier in this chapter.

How has your client changed behavior in the past?

- Increase your client's self-efficacy by discussing her past attempts at behavior change and identifying strategies that worked then and could help with increasing physical activity now (figure 7.2).
- Address any problems that have gotten in the way during past attempts at behavior change and may become an issue for changing physical activity (figure 7.5).

How might your client benefit from increasing physical activity?

- Ask your client to write down how she might benefit from increasing her physical activity (figure 7.3).
- Suggest some benefits your client may not have thought of yet or has not yet noticed.
- Encourage your client to learn more about these benefits and to look for additional benefits of increasing physical activity.
- Have your client assess how important these benefits are to her.

What might your client need to give up to become more physically active, and what barriers does your client need to address?

- Ask your client to write down what she would have to give up to increase physical activity and what she might find unpleasant about physical activity (figure 7.4).
- Have your client assess how difficult these things will be to give up.
- Help your client differentiate between true barriers and excuses.
- Help your client find solutions for these barriers using the IDEA approach (figure 7.5).

STAGE 3

How can you help your client to become more confident about physical activity?

- Let your client know that you believe in her ability to increase her physical activity.
- Emphasize that your client has already made progress because she is doing some physical activity.
- Work on increasing your client's confidence by pinpointing perceived obstacles and developing realistic strategies for overcoming them (figures 7.4 and 7.5).
- Relate your client's past successes at behavior change with her ability to become more physically active (figure 7.2).
- Discuss what went wrong during past attempts at behavior change and reframe them as learning experiences that can teach your client what to do differently this time around.
- Help your client to think about what she likes most and least about physical activity and how her activity plans can be modified to reflect these preferences.
- Encourage your client to think of herself as a physically active person.

What goals might help your client become more physically active?

- Work with your client to set manageable short- and long-term goals, perhaps around a mediator of behavior change (see chapter 4) that can help her increase her physical activity (figure 7.6).
- Create a plan for replacing 15 minutes of sedentary time during the week with some type of activity (substituting alternatives).
- Suggest that your client set a goal of asking a friend to join her for a 20-minute walk in the upcoming week (enlisting social support).
- Help your client think of a couple of ways to remind herself to be more active and suggest she try to implement them over the week (reminding oneself).
- Encourage your client to commit herself to increasing her daily activity by 5 more minutes over the next week (self-efficacy; committing oneself).
- Agree on something your client can do or a small gift she can buy herself to reward success in achieving her goals (rewarding oneself).
- Suggest that your client allow herself to engage in a pleasurable sedentary activity (e.g., watching a favorite movie, surfing the Web, taking a short nap) only after she has accomplished one of her activity goals.
- Set up a point system that your client can use to earn a larger reward (e.g., accomplishing a small goal earns 2 points; 30 accumulated points can be used to purchase a camping trip).
- Discuss what someone significant in your client's life might be able to do or say to reward your client's physical activity achievements (enlisting social support).

(continued) ▶

STAGE 3

Has your client succeeded in increasing physical activity?

■ Have your client keep a daily activity log to monitor her minutes of activity (figure 6.2).

■ Ask your client to write down the number of steps accumulated on a step counter over the course of the day (figures 6.5 and 6.6).

■ Reassess your client's stage of change (see chapter 2).

■ Consider giving your client the processes of change questionnaire (questionnaire 4.1 in appendix A) to see whether she is using more strategies for change.

■ Measure your client's confidence to see whether it has improved by using the self-efficacy questionnaire (questionnaire 4.2 in appendix A).

■ Administer the decisional balance questionnaire (questionnaire 4.4 in appendix A).

STAGE 4

DOING ENOUGH PHYSICAL ACTIVITY

Even though your client is physically active at the recommended level, his challenge is to maintain his physical activity over time. Here are some suggestions for using the strategies discussed in this chapter to help a client in this stage to make physical activity a habit.

Is it physically safe for your client to continue being physically active?

- Give your client the PAR-Q (figure 7.1) to assess any changes in health status relevant to physical activity.
- Refer your client to a physician if any health problems or discomforts related to activity arise.

How has your client changed behavior in the past?

- Discuss your client's past attempts at behavior change to identify strategies that he may not have applied yet to physical activity (figure 7.2).
- Address any problems that have gotten in the way during past attempts at behavior change and may be an issue for continuing physical activity (figure 7.5).

How has your client benefited from becoming physically active?

- Ask your client to write down how he has benefited from his physical activity (figure 7.3).
- Suggest some benefits your client may not have thought of yet or has not yet noticed.
- Encourage your client to learn more about the benefits of physical activity and to look for additional benefits as he continues to be physically active.
- Have your client assess how important these benefits are to him.

What are the costs of being physically active? What barriers might your client still need to address?

- Ask your client to write down what he has given up to become physically active and what he still finds unpleasant about physical activity (figure 7.4).
- Have your client assess how important these things are to him.
- Use the IDEA problem-solving approach to reduce any perceived costs and any remaining barriers (figure 7.5).
- Encourage your client to think about any obstacles that might arise in the future that could interfere with his ability to stay active. Create a plan for these potential problems.

(continued) ▶

STAGE 4 *(continued)*

How can your client become even more confident about physical activity?

▪ Discuss any negative thoughts concerning physical activity with which your client is still struggling and work on developing more positive thoughts.

▪ Help your client to think about what he likes most and least about physical activity. Find out what you can do to help make physical activity more enjoyable, convenient, or safe for your client.

▪ Work with your client to instill confidence that he can start up his physical activity program anew, if for some reason he should stop.

▪ Remind your client of how far he has come and praise him for his efforts.

What goals might help your client stay physically active?

▪ Help your client to generate short-term goals for physical activity or for mediators that may help him to sustain his motivation.

▪ Help your client decide on an appropriate amount of activity in a given week (committing oneself).

▪ Suggest that your client try a new activity (enjoyment).

▪ Encourage your client to ask someone to exercise with him (enlisting social support).

▪ Suggest that your client think of someone in his life for whom he can serve as a role model. Have your client commit to a behavior that might help motivate this person to become active (caring about consequences to others; committing oneself).

▪ Help your client to develop some long-term goals (committing oneself; see figure 7.6).

▪ Find a walking or running event or race that is going to take place in the community. Work on a plan for your client to train for this event (committing oneself).

▪ Set up a reward plan for your client's continued regular activity for the next month (rewarding oneself).

▪ Help your client decide on a number of miles to try to accumulate over the next 3 months (goal setting).

▪ Consult with a health professional, if necessary, to determine appropriate physiological goals for your client, such as decreasing cholesterol or blood pressure.

▪ Agree on a small gift your client can buy himself for accomplishing his goal (rewarding oneself).

▪ Suggest that your client allow himself to engage in a pleasurable sedentary activity (e.g., watching a favorite movie, surfing the Web, taking a short nap) only after he has accomplished one of his activity goals.

- Set up a point system that your client can use to earn a larger reward (e.g., accomplishing a small goal earns 2 points; 50 accumulated points can be used to purchase new walking shoes).

- Discuss what someone significant in your client's life might be able to do or say to reward your client's physical activity achievements (enlisting social support).

- Remind your client to review some of the benefits he has already achieved from physical activity. These benefits are natural rewards for exercising.

- Suggest that your client post some reminders in his environment so that he remembers to praise himself for his success (reminding oneself).

How can your client track success?

- Have your client keep a daily activity log to monitor his minutes of activity (figure 6.2).

- Ask your client to write down the number of steps accumulated on a step counter over the course of the day (see chapter 6). Develop a plan for your client to reward himself after he achieves a particular number.

- Suggest that your client monitor his resting heart rate or level of exertion during activity. Have him record them on a graph so he can see the changes over time.

- If your client has a short period of inactivity (as a result of work demands or illness) but then resumes activity following this episode, praise him for his ability to get back on track.

STAGE 4

STAGE 5

MAKING PHYSICAL ACTIVITY A HABIT

Your client is somewhat of a seasoned pro if she is in this stage. However, you can be beneficial to her by using the strategies discussed in this chapter to help her prepare for any future setbacks and help her increase her enjoyment of physical activity.

Is it physically safe for your client to continue being physically active?

- ▪ Give your client the PAR-Q (figure 7.1) to assess any changes in health status relevant to physical activity.
- ▪ Refer your client to a physician if any health problems arise.

How has your client changed behavior in the past?

- ▪ Discuss your client's past attempts at behavior change to identify strategies that she may not have applied yet to physical activity.
- ▪ Address any problems that have gotten in the way during past attempts at behavior change and may be an issue for continuing physical activity (figure 7.5).

How has your client benefited from continuing to be physically active?

- ▪ Suggest some benefits from physical activity that your client may not have noticed.
- ▪ Encourage your client to learn more about the benefits of physical activity.
- ▪ Encourage your client to periodically remind herself of how she benefits from continuing to be physically active; this helps to sustain motivation (figure 7.3).

What are the costs of being physically active? What barriers might your client still need to address?

- ▪ Ask your client to write down what she has given up to become physically active and what she still finds unpleasant about physical activity (figure 7.4).
- ▪ Have your client assess how important these things are to her.
- ▪ Use the IDEA problem-solving approach to further reduce any perceived costs (figure 7.5).
- ▪ Work with your client to come up with ways to increase her enjoyment of physical activity.
- ▪ Encourage your client to think about any obstacles that might arise in the future that could interfere with her ability to stay active. Help her create a plan for these potential problems.

How can your client maintain confidence about staying active over the long term?

- Explore with your client options for making activity more enjoyable.
- Work with your client to instill confidence that she can start up her physical activity program anew, if for some reason she should stop.
- Remind your client of how far she has come and praise her for her efforts.
- Remind your client of the benefits she has already achieved.
- Encourage your client to become a mentor to someone else who is trying to accomplish what she already has.

What goals might help your client stay physically active?

- Help your client to generate short-term goals to sustain her motivation (committing oneself; see figure 7.6).
- Suggest that your client try a new activity (enjoyment).
- Encourage your client to ask someone to be physically active with her (enlisting social support).
- Suggest that your client think of someone in her life for whom she can serve as a role model. Have your client commit to a behavior that might help motivate this person to become active (caring about consequences to others; committing oneself).
- Help your client to develop some long-term goals (committing oneself).
- Find a walking or running event or race that is going to take place in the community. Work on a plan for your client to train for this event (committing oneself).
- Set up a reward plan for your client's continued regular activity for the next month (rewarding oneself).
- Help your client decide on a number of miles to try to accumulate over the next 3 months (goal setting).
- Consult with a health professional, if necessary, to determine appropriate physiological goals for your client, such as decreasing cholesterol or blood pressure.
- Agree on a small gift your client can buy herself for accomplishing her goal (rewarding oneself).
- Suggest that your client allow herself to engage in some pleasurable sedentary activity (e.g., talking to a friend on the phone) only after she has accomplished one of her activity goals.
- Set up a point system that your client can use to earn a larger reward (e.g., accomplishing a small goal earns 2 points; 80 accumulated points can be used to purchase new exercise equipment).

(continued) ▷

STAGE 5

- Discuss what someone significant in your client's life might be able to do or say to reward her for her physical activity achievements (enlisting social support).

- Remind your client to look over some of the benefits she has already achieved from physical activity. These benefits are natural rewards for exercising.

- Suggest that your client post some reminders in her environment so that she remembers to praise herself for her success (reminding oneself).

How can your client track success?

- Have your client keep a daily activity log to monitor her minutes of activity (see figure 6.2).

- Ask your client to write down the number of steps accumulated on a step counter over the course of the day (see figure 6.5). Help your client develop a plan for rewarding herself after she achieves a particular number.

- Suggest that your client monitor resting heart rate (figure 6.7) or level of exertion during activity. Have her record these on a graph so she can see the changes over time.

- If your client has a short period of inactivity (as a result of work demands or illness) but then resumes activity following this episode, praise her for her ability to get back on track.

Conclusion

In this chapter we showed how the stages of change model can be applied to working with individuals. We shared the rationale and tools for assessing your client's physical and psychological readiness for physical activity. We also described the importance of your client's past experiences in making behavior changes and how this information can guide current plans for behavior change. Specific strategies for measuring your client's confidence and for goal setting were described. We also discussed the need to measure change in your client's behavior so as to empower her to continue the journey of behavior change and maintenance of that change.

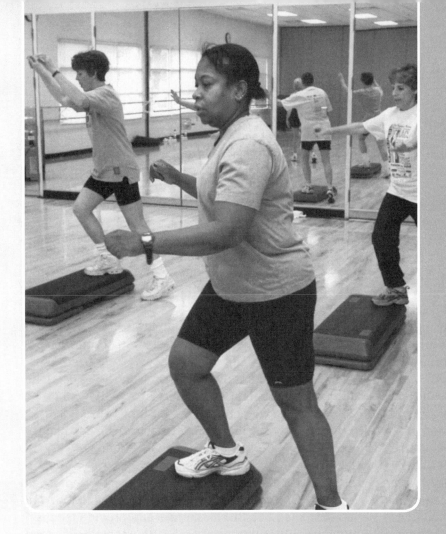

CHAPTER 8

Using the Stages Model in Group Counseling Programs

Many people have difficulty solving physical activity–related problems on their own. A group physical activity program can offer these people additional ideas about becoming more active through other group members' experiences and thoughts on the subject. Group physical activity programs provide additional channels of social support through relationships with group members and the group leader. Group members may choose to get together outside of the regular group time and thus provide each other with more regular support. The group leader can facilitate this by encouraging group members to share their phone numbers and call each other during tough times or for problem solving and support. Finally, group counseling has the benefit of being a cost- and time-effective way for health promoters to help several people at once.

Many types of groups promote physical activity. People engaging in physical activity in the same place, such as a gym or pool, and an instructor leading a group of people in an exercise class can both be considered group-based programs. Other groups are more accurately described as health educational because they offer health information related to physical activity. Still others provide both health education and specific skill-building strategies and behavioral techniques that apply psychological theory to behavior change. One example of such a program is Project Active, discussed in chapter 5 and also later in this chapter (Dunn et al., 1999). Then there are groups that are more psychotherapeutic in nature in that they help clients to explore personal habits, emotions, and relationships that affect physical activity habits and use interactions among group members to raise issues and provide feedback related to physical activity. Whether you create a health educational group, behavioral skill-building group, psychotherapeutic group, or group exercise class will depend on the setting in which you work, your professional training, your style as a group leader, and the needs of your clients. Our purpose in this chapter is to discuss strategies for incorporating the stages of motivational readiness for change model in group programs that teach members behavioral skills that allow them to be more active outside of group sessions and to incorporate physical activity into their daily lives.

Leading a Stage-Based Group

Group programs are influenced by group members' stages of motivational readiness for change and by the role and teaching style of the group leader (Rinne & Toropainen, 1998). You are the group leader presumably because you possess information and expertise that your clients do not. Therefore, one of your roles is to provide information that you have gained in your professional training. You are likely to adopt the role of *teacher* and use a didactic leadership style more often with clients who are in the earlier stages of motivational readiness (stage 1, not thinking about change, and stage 2, thinking about change). For clients in stage 2, thinking about change, and stage 3, doing some physical activity, you may find yourself being a *motivator,* who encourages them to try new skills. For clients in stages 3 (doing some activity) and 4 (doing enough activity), you can also be less didactic and serve more as a *facilitator,* who encourages group members to share ideas, experiences, and support. For clients in the later stages, 4 and 5 (doing enough physical activity and making physical activity a habit, respectively), you will probably find that you need to give even less information but rather serve as an *analyzer,* who helps clients identify potential pitfalls, and as a *consultant,* who offers suggestions for avoiding pitfalls or handling them better. As the group leader, you will also need to be flexible about your role and instructional style when the people in your group are at different stages of motivational readiness for change (Rinne & Toropainen, 1998). Table 8.1 describes teaching styles and instructor roles suited to each of the stages of motivational readiness.

Setting Up a Stage-Based Group

There are no hard-and-fast rules about the number of people you should have in a group or the number of sessions you should hold. Groups with fewer members offer more opportunity for participation and instructor attention. Larger groups, on the other hand, are more cost- and time-effective. Both issues are important to keep in mind when deciding the size of a group. Our general guideline is to have a maximum of 15 people if there is to be individual participation. Five people is probably the minimum useful number for idea sharing and discussions among the participants. That way, if one or two people are unable to attend a given session, enough members will still be present to exchange thoughts and ideas.

Rinne and Toropainen (1998) suggested that two or three group sessions are not likely to have much impact, whereas group sessions that stretch over several months may become boring. Ten to 12 weekly group sessions are appropriate for group treatment. If the group expresses an interest in continuing to meet, consider having a break at the end of 12 weeks or so and then scheduling a follow-up group in 1 month so that members can share their experiences of continuing their activity plans on their own (Rinne & Toropainen, 1998).

If you will be leading a larger group, consider having a colleague serve as a coleader. It is always nice to have more than one professional perspective and to share the work of preparing for group, facilitating group discussions, and writing chart notes afterward if your setting requires you to do so. If group members are in various stages of motivational readiness and you decide to break them up into smaller groups based on stage, each coleader can take responsibility for facilitating a subgroup.

Consider calling participants who do not show up for a group session or two. Giving no-shows a quick call helps with accountability and lets them know that you missed their presence in the group. It also gives you a chance to learn whether something about the group made them decide not to attend

TABLE 8.1   Group Leader's Role and Teaching Style in a Stage-Based Group

Stage	Leader's role	Teaching style	Sample input
1: Not thinking about change	Teacher	Share information	"Let me share with you some ways that physical activity might benefit you, some of which you may not have thought about."
2: Thinking about change	Teacher	Share information	"Research studies have shown that taking a 10-minute walk has important health benefits."
	Motivator	Provide encouragement, increase confidence	"To start out, just do what you feel comfortable with, such as a 5- or 10-minute walk. You sound ready to move on to this step."
3: Doing some activity	Teacher	Share information	"One of the most helpful ways of making activity a part of your life is to monitor your progress and to give yourself rewards. Let me share with you some ways you might go about doing this."
	Motivator	Provide encouragement	"You are making great progress. You should reward yourself for all your hard work."
	Facilitator	Promote group process (e.g., idea sharing and support among group members)	"What strategies have others tried for fitting in physical activity during a hectic day?"
4: Doing enough activity	Facilitator	Promote group process	"Let's all brainstorm some ideas for what to tell yourself when you don't feel motivated."
	Analyzer	Help identify potential pitfalls	"I've noticed that you really enjoy outdoor activities. Any thoughts on what you are going to do this fall when the weather gets colder?"
	Consultant	Suggest strategies for preventing relapse (e.g., avoiding pitfalls, better handling of pitfalls)	"It sounds like activity is one of the first things to go when you have a lot on your plate. One thing others have found helpful is to try being active first thing in the morning rather than waiting until after work when they are tired and need to take care of their families. Let's talk about how you might do this."

Stage	Leader's role	Teaching style	
5: Making activity a habit	Motivator	Provide encouragement	"You are active at the level recommended by health experts and have been able to keep it up. Even though you may not be an athlete or a 'hard-core' exerciser, I hope you think of yourself as an active person."
	Facilitator	Promote group process	"Why don't we go around the room and say what strategies have been most helpful for keeping active over the long term."
	Analyzer	Help identify potential pitfalls	"It seems that many of you have found an activity or two that you really enjoy. This is great, but one thing we worry about is people's becoming bored with the same routine over time. Let's discuss ways to prevent this."
	Consultant	Suggest strategies for preventing relapse	"Have you thought about what you would do if you were to stop being active for a while? This is bound to happen, and it's important to have a backup plan to keep this from making you stop being active altogether."

Reprinted from *Patient Education and Counseling*, Vol. 33, R. Rinne and E. Toropainen, "How to lead a group-practical," S69-S76, Copyright 1998, with permission from Elsevier Science.

or whether personal circumstances kept them from coming. Sometimes people drop out because they believe they are not making progress. A quick phone call to these people gives you an opportunity to reiterate that people's stages of readiness to make a personal behavior change vary and that attending group sessions should be considered progress in itself. You could also encourage the client to consider one or two individual sessions, if available, to get him back on track before, or in addition to, rejoining the group. Whatever your policy is on missed sessions, tell the people in your group what it is at the outset so that they know what to expect.

Defining Individual Goals

As a group instructor, you will be trying to work on the goals of each individual within the group, which can be challenging if the members of your group are at different stages in the change continuum. For instance, one member may have the personal goal of being active at least 5 days a week for 30 to 45 minutes at a time. Another member might be satisfied if she maintains 3 days of activity on a steady basis. For a third group member, trying one 10-minute brisk walk at some point during the course of the group will be a significant achievement. One way to handle individual goal setting when members are at different stages of motivational readiness is to encourage members in stages 1 and 2 to set mainly process-oriented goals while members in stages 3, 4, and 5 can be encouraged to set both process-oriented and physical activity behavior goals.

By process goals, we are referring to behaviors other than actual physical activity behavior that can help a person move along the stage continuum, such as reading about the benefits of physical activity, asking someone to be a walking partner, or finding a location to try a different type of physical activity (e.g., a large, empty parking lot to try in-line skating for the first time, parks with good hiking trails). Too often individuals and exercise promoters focus mainly on the physical activity behavior goals and place much less (or no) emphasis on process goals. As a result, people in the earlier stages drop out because they are not ready to set physical activity goals. Process goals also make good homework assignments to do between formal group sessions.

Physical activity goals are related to the frequency, duration, intensity, and type of actual physical activity behaviors (e.g., taking three 15-minute brisk walks during a given week, maintaining 150 minutes of moderate-intensity physical activity per week for the next 2 months). In your role of group leader, you should help group members to set both short- and long-term goals related to their physical activity per week behavior (see figure 7.6 in chapter 7 for a form that can be used for this purpose). You might define short-term goals as those that group members can accomplish in the week between group sessions, whereas long-term goals are those they can accomplish by the end of the group program. Walking a predetermined distance (e.g., across the state), becoming fit enough to participate in a community walk, and achieving enough reward points to cash in for a weekend away are examples of long-term goals.

Regardless of the type of goal, encourage each group member to set goals that are both *realistic* and *evaluative*. By realistic we mean that goals should be challenging yet attainable and thus enhance clients' confidence in their ability to be active. By evaluative we mean that goals should be articulated in such a way that the client and others can observe whether the outcome has been achieved. A client will have difficulty determining whether he has achieved a goal of becoming healthier, but he can determine that he is able to walk farther or that his cholesterol level has dropped from 220 to 200. Working on goal setting in a group setting is a great way to teach this important skill. Group members can learn from each other how to articulate an activity goal in such a way that it can be observed and measured, and they can get ideas for their own goals as they listen to others.

Setting goals also provides a format that you can use to structure a standard group session. The following is a suggested format that you can use for each group session:

- Assess how group members did with their individual short-term goals over the past week and assess their progress toward their long-term goals.
- Present the topic for the current group session.
- Evaluate whether group members obtained the information they needed or hoped to receive, and if you, as the group leader, covered all the information you had intended to convey for that session.
- Have each member set a short-term physical activity or behavioral goal for the upcoming week.

To give you an idea of how a stage-based physical activity group might work, we discuss in the next section a program that provided stage-based behavioral skills training in a group format. A sample of the curriculum used in Project Active is in table 8.2.

Learning from a Sample Stage-Based Curriculum

Project Active (Dunn et al., 1997; Dunn et al., 1998) was a study that compared a traditional, structured, gymnasium-based exercise program with a lifestyle program that emphasized the newer physical activity recommendation to accumulate moderate-intensity activities on 5 or more days of the week (Haskell et al., 2007). Both programs had a 6-month intensive intervention phase and an 18-month follow-up intervention phase (Dunn et al., 1999). Participants were in either stage 2 or stage 3 at the beginning of the program. For the first 6 months, the lifestyle program was delivered as a group program in which about 15 participants at a time met with group facilitators who had training in psychology, health education, or exercise science for 1 hour, 1 night a week for the first 4 months and then every other week for 2 more months. Meeting topics revolved around cognitive and behavioral skill building, developing self-efficacy for physical activity, and solving problems and focusing on the individual issues of both group members and facilitators. The goal was to help participants learn skills to enable them to integrate activities of at least moderate intensity into their daily lives. As self-efficacy and use of the cognitive and behavioral skills increased, the program tapered to fewer group meetings (monthly and then bimonthly) throughout the remainder of the 2-year program.

The lifestyle approach was based on the stages of motivational readiness for change (Prochaska & DiClemente, 1983) and social cognitive theory (Bandura, 1986, 1997). At the outset of this program, participants were assessed and told their stage of motivational readiness (e.g., stage 2, thinking about change). Each month for the next 6 months, their motivational readiness for physical activity was assessed, and they were given a stage-matched physical

TABLE 8.2   **Lifestyle Curriculum and Targeted Behavioral and Cognitive Strategies**

Week	Session title and group activity	Behavioral and cognitive processes
1	Getting to Know You—Monitoring sedentary pursuits, substituting active alternatives	Increasing knowledge, substituting alternatives
2	Understanding Barriers—Listing personal barriers and benefits, fitting short bouts of activity into daily life	Comprehending benefits, increasing healthy opportunities
3	Learning More—Setting goals, assessing enjoyable physical activities, demonstrating energy intensity	Increasing knowledge
4	Enlisting Aid—Identifying social support sources and types of support	Enlisting social support, committing yourself
5	Getting Confidence—Reflecting on overcoming barriers, problem solving to overcome obstacles	Increasing self-efficacy
6	Scavenging for Physical Activity—Examining alternative, nontraditional ways to be physically active	Increasing healthy opportunities, substituting alternatives
7	Rewarding Yourself—Choosing appropriate rewards for reaching short- and long-term goals	Rewarding yourself, committing yourself
8	Time Management—Prioritizing daily activities to fit in physical activity	Decision making, increasing healthy opportunities
9	Scouting Physical Activity in Your Community—Using maps and resource guides to find new activities	Increasing healthy opportunities, enlisting social support
10	Reviewing Goals—Using a step counter to monitor activity and set goals	Reminding yourself
11	Physical Activity Fair—Discussing and demonstrating favorite physical activities	Committing yourself, increasing self-efficacy
12	Cognitive Restructuring and Relapse Prevention—Learning how to change all-or-none thinking, planning for relapses	Substituting alternatives, comprehending benefits

activity manual shown to be effective at enhancing physical activity behavior (Marcus et al., 1992; Marcus, Bock, et al., 1998; Marcus, Emmons, et al., 1998; Marcus, Lewis, et al., 2007; Marcus, Napolitano, et al., 2007).

Participants were also informed that their program goal was to accumulate at least 30 minutes of moderate-intensity activity on most days of the week (Pate et al., 1995; USDHHS, 1996). Participants were instructed to tell program staff their individual goals for becoming more physically active.

Creating Change Through Group Counseling

Sam, a 48-year-old engineer, was encouraged by his wife to participate in the Project Active study because he had complained of having less energy and more trouble sleeping over the past year. Sam was pleased to be assigned to the lifestyle group because he knew he would not like attending a gym on a regular basis. However, at first Sam was skeptical about how much the lifestyle curriculum and group support could help him because he had such a busy work and personal schedule.

When Sam attended his first group session, he was in stage 3 (doing some physical activity), had low self-efficacy for physical activity, identified several barriers that prevented him from being physically active (lack of time being the primary one), and had made few steps toward becoming more active to date. However, Sam did play golf every Sunday, weather permitting, and he carried his clubs when he played. During the first group session, Sam reported that he saw no way to add physical activity during his workweek because of work demands, and he had no time to add activity on Saturdays because this was his wife's day to do errands and spend time with friends (Sunday was his day to do things on his own). The group leader encouraged Sam to think about adding physical activity in different ways, rather than thinking of adding another long bout of activity similar to his Sunday golf game. The group leader encouraged Sam to think about how he could fit in short bouts of activity during his workday. Sam agreed to think about this. In subsequent group sessions he listened as other group members shared some strategies that were working for them. Although Sam continued to assert that he could not change his workweek, he did begin to think that there might be a way for him to get in some activity on a regular basis without having to change his workweek.

Sam began to think about the fact that he often got distracted if he sat in front of his computer for more than an hour at a time. In fact, he admitted that after every hour of sitting he "lost" the next 15 minutes zoning out before he could get back on track. By week 6 of the program Sam decided that he would try setting his watch to go off every hour on the hour. If he was sitting at his desk, he would get up and take a 2-minute walk. During the next week he found he could easily take three 2-minute walks per day. Although he saw no increase in his productivity as a result, he also realized he did not lose any productivity despite these 6 minutes of walking per day.

With the support of two other men with busy schedules who were in the group, over the next 8 weeks Sam first increased the number of times per day he took hourly walks, and then he increased the number of minutes of some of the walks. As a result, 4 months into the program, on a typical workday, Sam was taking two 2-minute walks, two 5-minute walks, and two 10-minute walks. He found that not only did he not lose any productivity, but he actually was more productive during his 10-hour workday as a result of these walking breaks. Moreover, he was now getting in at least 30 minutes of moderate-intensity physical activity most days of the week, and still playing golf on Sunday. Best of all, his wife said he was less irritable with the kids and more engaged in family dinner time conversation! Sam was now in stage 4 (doing enough physical activity), and he was optimistic that he could sustain this new habit.

Incorporated into the lifestyle group meetings curriculum were the 10 processes of change, self-efficacy, and decision making for physical activity (see chapters 2, 3, and 4), which are part of the stages of motivational readiness for change model (Prochaska & DiClemente, 1983) and social cognitive theory (Bandura, 1986, 1997) that can be applied to physical activity adoption and maintenance. These ideas were the basis of the strategies for building self-efficacy and cognitive and behavioral skills. For example, increasing knowledge is one of the five cognitive processes of change and can include increasing knowledge about the importance of physical activity and increasing knowledge about one's own sedentary habits. During one of the first lifestyle group meetings, participants were asked to complete a 1-week log of the time they spent sitting. At the next session, they shared their results with the group, and each person developed a plan within the context of their stage of motivational readiness and life circumstance to decrease the amount of time spent sitting as illustrated in the case example on page 117. Samples of activities from the 6-month curriculum and the corresponding psychological processes are shown in table 8.2. The full curriculum is available in the book *Active Living Every Day* (Blair, Dunn, Marcus, Carpenter, & Jaret, 2001).

Assessing Your Effectiveness as a Leader

To determine whether you, as the group leader, achieved your objective for a session or topic, you can use group discussion, such as reviewing information provided in group meetings and how participants have applied various concepts and strategies. You might also consider obtaining more formal feedback by administering questionnaires or having group members fill out written evaluations to help you determine if they consider the information covered in group discussion useful. If the topic of the session was self-efficacy, you might want to have participants complete the confidence (self-efficacy) questionnaire found in appendix A at the beginning of the session so that they can identify areas in which they are more or less confident. Then, after spending the session discussing ways to stay active in challenging situations such as vacations and bad weather, you might have them fill out the questionnaire again to see whether there have been any improvements in self-efficacy. If there is no standardized measure available for the topic you covered, you can have participants answer a few questions on the content you covered to see how well they learned the information.

You do not necessarily have to collect participants' responses to questionnaires or questions; this exercise could just be a way for participants to collect information about themselves. If you do decide to collect their answers, you may opt to have them respond anonymously so that their answers are more honest. Alternatively, you could have group members put their names on the questionnaires and then write out specific feedback for participants to read and consider privately or write down ways they might want to try to increase confidence in the areas in which they are struggling.

You may also want to encourage group members to keep diaries between group sessions to track their progress and to jot down issues as they arise for discussion at the next group. Some examples of useful content to include in a physical activity diary are provided in chapter 6 (see figures 6.1, 6.3, and 6.5 on pages 66, 69, and 73).

Stage-Specific Suggestions for Group Activities

In this section we provide some strategies that you can incorporate into your own group curriculum. You can select among the options based on the stages of motivational readiness of your participants. If your group consists mainly of people who are in the same or similar stages of change, you might use the strategies described under the appropriate stage. If you find that your group has members in both the earliest stages (i.e., 1 or 2) and the later stages (i.e., 4 or 5), you might find it easier to break the group into smaller subgroups to adequately address the needs of each member. We would also encourage you to come up with your own ideas for group activities based on your setting and the needs of your clients.

STAGE 1

NOT THINKING ABOUT CHANGE

You may find that some of the people in this earliest stage are enrolled in your group but are not interested in considering physical activity at the present time. Perhaps they joined to please someone else such as a physician or family member. Or, maybe they initially joined the group because they were in stage 2 or 3 but then regressed to an earlier stage during the course of the group. Let them know that they can still attend the group meetings even if they are not interested in starting activity right now, because they may get some ideas that will be helpful if they should want to be active later on. Some of the following strategies may encourage them to think about trying physical activity again or perhaps for the first time.

What might you do to keep these people involved in your group?

- Determine their willingness to participate in discussions or do other behavioral assignments such as looking up the benefits of physical activity.
- Lead a discussion about how people's sedentary behavior might affect those around them.
- Discuss another relevant health behavior (e.g., smoking cessation, healthy eating) and relate physical activity to this behavior.
- Discuss past attempts at becoming physically active. Is this related to why they are not interested in change now?
- Ask if you can check in with them every month or so to see where they are with physical activity.

(continued) ▶

STAGE 1 (continued)

- Foster social support from other group members for those who are still attending the group meetings even though they are not thinking about becoming physically active now.
- Ask them to list any barriers to physical activity.
- Administer the PAR-Q (found in figure 7.1) and address health events that might preclude physical activity.
- Lead a group discussion on true barriers versus excuses.
- Consider addressing body image. Listen for any clues that suggest that some members are resistant to becoming physically active because they are embarrassed by how they would look engaged in physical activity.
- Ask them what they would need to consider doing physical activity.
- Present recommended levels of physical activity and the benefits that can be gained through accumulated moderate-intensity physical activities.
- List lifestyle activities that can help them achieve health benefits if performed at a moderate intensity (see chapter 6 for ideas). Notions such as "no pain, no gain" may be leading some to remain at this stage.
- Invite a guest speaker to give a presentation on the benefits of physical activity.
- Consider some goals that might help these people move toward considering change.
- Reinforce the idea that achieving other behavioral or cognitive goals, even if they do not include actual physical activity, is productive and worthwhile.
- Ask these group members to think about a behavior, other than physical activity, that they were successful at changing and generate a list of strategies that were helpful in these past attempts. You can write them on a blackboard or a big sheet of paper to help others get ideas for physical activity behavior change (figure 7.2).
- Ask group members to generate a list of common negative thoughts concerning physical activity and identify alternative positive thoughts they could use to replace them.

STAGE 2

THINKING ABOUT CHANGE

Group members in stage 2 are thinking about becoming more active and will probably find support from other group members helpful in their efforts to move toward actually trying this new behavior. Ideas from other group members who are participating in physical activity can help members in stage 2 to carefully plan their initial attempts at physical activity so that the experience is pleasant enough to try it again. Here are some ideas for helping group members who are thinking about change.

What information might help these group members to consider trying some physical activity?

- Present physical activity recommendations and the benefits that can be gained from accumulating moderate-intensity physical activities.
- List lifestyle activities that can help them achieve health benefits if performed at a moderate intensity. Notions such as "no pain, no gain" may be preventing some from becoming physically active (see chapter 6).
- Present various types of social support (described in chapter 4). Have each participant identify areas in which social support would be helpful in getting started.
- Invite a guest speaker to give a presentation on the benefits of physical activity.
- Lead a discussion about how their sedentary behavior might affect those around them.
- Discuss another relevant health behavior (e.g., smoking cessation, healthy eating) and relate physical activity to this behavior.
- Ask them to list barriers to physical activity.
- Use the IDEA approach described in chapter 7 to teach group members how to overcome perceived barriers. Have group members practice this problem-solving approach with each other or on their own (see figure 7.5).
- Consider addressing body image during one of the groups. Listen for any clues that suggest that some members have put off becoming physically active because they are embarrassed by how they would look engaged in physical activity.
- Discuss past attempts at becoming physically active. Is this related to why some group members are not physically active now or have low confidence?
- Lead a group discussion on true barriers versus excuses for not trying physical activity.
- Lead a group discussion on priority setting and where beginning physical activity fits in their list of priorities.
- Ask participants to list activities that might help them get started.

(continued) ▶

STAGE 2 *(continued)*

- Set up teams to investigate various aspects of physical activity (e.g., benefits of cardiorespiratory activities, benefits of weight training, mental health benefits of physical activity, local places to go swing dancing).

- Through group discussion, develop strategies for obtaining social support and rewarding others who provide social support.

- Ask group members to generate a list of common negative thoughts concerning physical activity. Have each group member identify an alternative positive thought that could replace each negative thought. For this activity, it is important that each person identify an alternative statement that will work for him or her.

- Discuss activities that people in stage 2 might like to try or find enjoyable.

- Encourage group members to plan when, where, and with whom they might try some of these activities.

- Think of ways in which some light activities can be stepped up a notch into moderate-intensity activities (see chapter 6). To accomplish this, the leader could ask participants to brainstorm ideas or the leader could provide examples to the group.

- Post the commit dates for trying a physical activity on a bulletin board or on a handout.

- Consider goals that might help these participants move toward considering change. Doing this in group discussion can be greatly beneficial because one participant can learn from another. Stating goals and publicly committing to plans to meet said goals can enable group members to provide suggestions for helping others reach their goals.

- Ask group members to talk to someone they know who was successful at becoming physically active and get that person's advice. Have them share this advice with each other at the next meeting.

- Have each group member complete a personal time study to monitor the time spent sitting and the time spent engaging in some physical activity during two typical weekdays and a typical weekend day (see chapter 6). Spend part of the next group meeting brainstorming ideas for decreasing sedentary time and increasing time spent in physical activity.

- Ask group members to look up information about physical activity and its benefits or discover interesting Web sites about physical activity as a homework assignment. Have the group members take turns reporting their findings at the next meeting.

- Plan a 10-minute walk either during group time or for participants to try on their own during the next week.

STAGE 3

DOING SOME PHYSICAL ACTIVITY

Participants in this stage are doing some physical activity but not enough. Group discussion that provides these people with additional ideas and strategies for increasing their activity level will be helpful, as will support from other group members. Be sure to encourage goal setting for both behavioral skills and actual physical activity behaviors. Here are some ideas for group members in this stage.

What are the remaining barriers?

▪ Choose an obstacle that is interfering with physical activity for one or several of the group members. Demonstrate how to use the IDEA approach described in chapter 7 to develop potential solutions for overcoming this barrier. Practice with other obstacles.

▪ Give a presentation on time management.

▪ Lead a group discussion on true barriers versus excuses for not increasing physical activity.

▪ Provide information that might help to increase physical activity.

▪ Discuss how to make small environmental changes (e.g., move home exercise equipment from a seldom-used spare bedroom to the room where the TV is located) that can help to promote physical activity.

▪ Teach group members strategies for incorporating short bouts of physical activity into their daily lives.

▪ Demonstrate energy intensity (see chapter 6), such as demonstrating brisk walking rather than casual walking.

▪ Work with group members on setting appropriate goals for gradually increasing their physical activity.

▪ Present various types of social support (described in chapter 4). Have each participant identify areas in which social support would be helpful in becoming more active. Through group discussion, develop strategies for obtaining social support and rewarding others who provide social support.

▪ Generate a list of rewards for achieving personal goals. Also, describe how one might use a point system to reward progress over time.

▪ Invite a guest speaker to give a presentation on the benefits of increasing physical activity.

▪ Describe how some light activities can be stepped up a notch to moderate-intensity activities (see chapter 6).

▪ Help participants generate a list of the kinds of activities that might help increase physical activity.

(continued) ▶

STAGE 3

- Have group members generate a list of common negative thoughts that interfere with physical activity. Have each group member identify an alternative positive self-statement that promotes physical activity to replace a negative thought that serves as an excuse to not be active.

- Use the group time to have participants complete the processes of change questionnaire found in appendix A. Give group members additional time to identify additional change strategies and get feedback from others on how they could implement these strategies.

- Have group members brainstorm ways they might remind themselves to be more active.

- Lead a group discussion on priority setting and where increasing physical activity fits in participants' list of priorities.

- Lead a discussion on the goals that might help an individual in stage 3 to increase physical activity participation.

- Ask group members to talk to someone they know who was successful at becoming regularly active and get that person's advice. Have them share this advice with each other at the next meeting.

- Have each group member complete a personal time study to monitor the time spent sitting and the time spent engaging in some physical activity during two typical weekdays and one typical weekend day (see chapter 6). Spend the next group meeting brainstorming ideas for decreasing sedentary time and increasing time spent in physical activity.

- Encourage group members to try a new type of physical activity.

- Have some group members give short presentations on the activities they like to do.

- Encourage short-term physical activity goals that are realistic and manageable. For example, people in stage 3 might consider increasing their current duration of physical activity per day by 5 or 10 minutes or their frequency of physical activity by 1 day.

STAGE 4

STAGE 4

DOING ENOUGH PHYSICAL ACTIVITY

Even though group members in stage 4 are physically active at the recommended level, their challenge will be to maintain physical activity over time. They will still benefit from information you present to them and from setting both behavioral and physical activity goals. Here are some suggestions for helping regularly active group members keep it up.

What information might help these participants stick with physical activity until it is a habit?

- Encourage group members to share ideas on alternative activities to help prevent boredom.

- Lead a discussion on how others can unintentionally (or intentionally) sabotage their best efforts to stay active. How have others overcome this issue?

- Discuss how group members have encouraged others to be appropriately supportive.

- Invite a guest lecturer to talk about or demonstrate a new type of activity such as tai chi, yoga, or kickboxing.

- Pass out information on local hiking or biking trails.

- Discuss ways to monitor activity such as activity logs, perceived exertion, or heart rate (see chapter 6).

- Explain the importance of rewarding oneself for accomplishing personal goals.

- Discuss common obstacles that can arise and get even the most dedicated exercisers off track (see chapter 7).

- Suggest the use of a step counter to monitor activity and set goals (see chapter 6). Bring one in and demonstrate how to set, wear, and read it. Present various ways to use the step counter for setting goals and monitoring progress.

- Invite a guest speaker to give a presentation on the benefits of regular physical activity.

- Teach group members strategies for incorporating short bouts of physical activity into their daily lives.

- Discuss the kinds of goals that might help maintain physical activity.

- Try a new activity as a group (e.g., ice skating at a nearby rink).

- Encourage group members to identify a role model who helps to motivate them.

- Have group members generate a personal list of rewards.

(continued) ▶

STAGE 4 *(continued)*

■ Ask group members to generate a list of what they have given up to become physically active or what they still find unpleasant about physical activity. Discuss ways to address these issues.

■ Work on appropriate goal setting to maintain motivation over the long term.

■ Go around the room and have participants say what types of benefits they believe they have already achieved. What benefits are they still working toward?

■ Problem-solve around any remaining obstacles some group members may still be experiencing.

■ Have group members brainstorm ways they might post reminders in their environments that encourage them to praise themselves for their success.

STAGE 5

MAKING PHYSICAL ACTIVITY A HABIT

Participants in stage 5 are quite knowledgeable about physical activity. However, group meetings can still be a valuable source of support and a forum for getting additional ideas. Having booster sessions once a month or so may remind stage 5 people to review what has helped them remain active, encourage them to think of new ways to keep activity enjoyable, and formulate a plan for any future setbacks. Here are some ideas for group activities relevant to those who have managed to keep active over time.

What kind of group activities might foster continued physical activity maintenance?

- Encourage group members to share ideas on alternative activities to help prevent boredom.
- Invite a guest lecturer to talk about or demonstrate a new type of activity such as spinning, cross-country skiing, or in-line skating.
- Try a new activity as a group (e.g., rock climbing at an indoor facility).
- Pass out information on local hiking or biking trails.
- Discuss ways to monitor activity (see chapter 6).
- Explain the importance of continuing to reward oneself for achieving personal goals. Have group members generate a personal list of rewards. Be sure to describe how one might use a point system to reward progress over time.
- Emphasize the importance of appropriate goal setting to maintain motivation over the long term.
- Spend time identifying possible setbacks and developing plans to prepare for and overcome them.
- Have participants try to think of alternative, nontraditional ways to be active.
- Encourage participants to become physical activity mentors to people they know who are less active.
- Discuss how members can change all-or-none thinking should they find themselves getting off track.
- Ask these group members to generate a list of what they have given up to remain physically active or what they still find unpleasant about physical activity. Discuss ways to address these issues.

STAGE 5

Conclusion

Although tailoring a program based on clients' stages of motivational readiness seems like an individual approach for promoting physical activity, it can be successfully used in a group setting, as this chapter describes. Your role as the group leader will vary depending on the stages of motivational readiness of your group members. The goals that you set for your group and for each individual in the group will also vary according to participants' stages of motivational readiness. Project Active is an example of a curriculum that was built around the stages of change and the processes of change. Leading a physical activity group program can be a fun and effective way of sharing ideas and supporting your clients in their efforts to be more physically active.

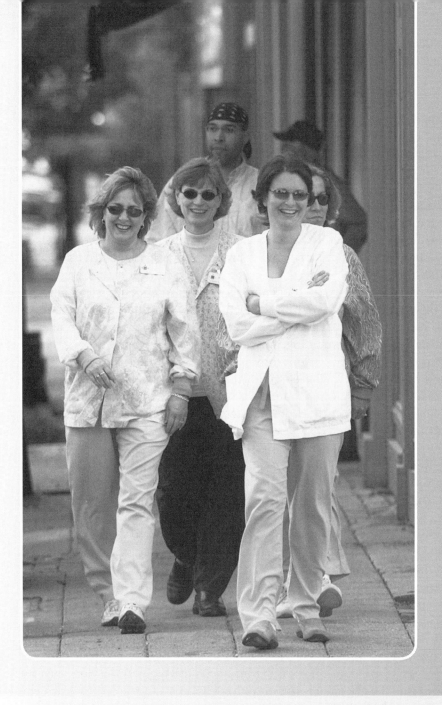

CHAPTER 9

Using the Stages Model in Work Site Programs

Between 110 and 115 million Americans go to work each day, and this number is estimated to increase to between 141 and 153 million people by the year 2010 (USDHHS, 1993). Workplace physical activity programs offer great opportunities for helping a lot of sedentary people become more active. Many people believe that the hours they spend at work interfere with the time they have available for physical activity. This does not have to be the case. In fact, interventions conducted in the workplace can be quite effective in increasing physical activity (Chan, Ryan, & Tudor-Locke, 2004; Marshall, Owen, & Bauman, 2004; Proper, Hildebrandt, Van der Beek, Twisk, & Van Mechelen, 2003).

The work setting can be an ideal place for disseminating physical activity–related information. Office settings typically have communication channels in place, such as voice mail, computer networks, newsletters, and mailboxes that can be useful for providing information about the benefits of physical activity or physical activity opportunities. In other workplaces, such as factories and retail settings, where employees may not have access to computer networks or voice mail, other channels such as paycheck stuffers and bulletin boards can be used to get the word out about physical activity programs you are offering.

Work environments can be arranged to provide opportunities for physical activity. Reminders to use the stairwell instead of the elevator can be posted, walking routes both inside the building and outside on the grounds can be marked and measured, and exercise equipment and facilities can even be provided. Furthermore, the workday actually provides hidden opportunities for activity so that employees can go home having already accumulated 30 minutes. Using coffee breaks to take 5- or 10-minute walks, holding one-on-one meetings while walking, and using the stairs instead of the elevator are examples of how this can be done. Finally, many work sites offer built-in social support networks that you can use to spread your message and support employees in their efforts to be more active.

Despite their proven value, work site physical activity programs traditionally recruit only about 20 percent of employees (Wanzel, 1994). This figure drops to only 10 percent after taking into account typical dropout rates for such programs. Furthermore, the employees who are attracted to work site programs tend to be the people who are already active to some degree (Marshall, Owen, & Bauman, 2004; Sharratt & Cox, 1988; Shephard, 1992).

Work site programs based on the stages of motivational readiness for change model take a proactive stance by attempting to reach even those who are not interested in making behavior change in the foreseeable future. Such programs, which foster a positive attitude toward physical activity and create a social norm that supports good health and positive health habits, may move the most unmotivated people closer to adopting some physical activity or at least thinking about becoming more active in the near future (USDHHS et al., 1999). These employees may later decide to participate in activity either at home or at other facilities in the community. This chapter discusses general issues regarding the stage-matched approach for work site programs and strategies that can be implemented in stage-matched workplace interventions.

Building Support for Your Program

Before you begin developing and implementing your work site program, you are obviously going to need to consider the employer's commitment to your efforts. For example, if you want employees to participate in assessments of motivational readiness while at work, then managerial support for using work time for this purpose is clearly necessary. Selling your program to the employer by explaining the benefits of increasing the mental and physical well-being of the staff is well worth your time and effort.

In a program we recently implemented simultaneously at a U.S. work site and an Australian work site, recruitment and retention of employees was dramatically better at the Australian work site. The primary reason was that the Australian CEO supported the program and told employees that he thought reading through the materials and thinking about becoming more active were good uses of their time. If you do not have the support of high-level management, you can still accomplish important goals in a work site program. You just may need more modest goals (e.g., increasing awareness about your intervention versus actual behavior change), and you need to make it clear to employees that you are delivering a home-based program through their workplace. In other words, instead of using work time to participate in the physical activity program, employees will receive the information during the work day but will read the information and work on increasing their activity outside of work hours.

Assessing Motivational Readiness

To target your physical activity program to employees based on their stages of motivational readiness for change, you need a means of assessment that is quick and easy for both the employees and the program administrators. Questionnaire 2.1 in appendix A can be answered quickly, and scoring it takes little time. It is also easy to train someone to do the scoring. However, in a pilot work site project we conducted, we found that written assessments were often lost in piles of paper on employees' desks or left at home. Also, employees became less interested in the program in the few days it took us to receive their questionnaires by interoffice mail and then send out stage-matched materials. Asking the five stage-determining questions by phone proved to be worth the extra effort in our program. Once we determined an employee's stage of readiness for change over the phone, we sent out the stage-matched materials to arrive the next day. Although this direct contact required extra time on our part and was more troublesome, we believe that it helped to engage employees in the program. In work settings where employees do not have private access to telephones, you could provide a convenience box on site into which employees could drop a short questionnaire, thus minimizing the delay for delivering stage-targeted materials.

If some component of your program requires registration, such as a seminar or skills-building class, consider putting questionnaire 2.1 on the registration form so that you can match the message delivered during the event. If your program does not require registration, consider having employees complete the stage-assessing questions as a way of entering a prize drawing (Glaros, 1997). Because entering the drawing does not necessarily commit the employee to the physical activity program, this is a good way to get a fairly accurate idea of where employees lie on the stages of change continuum.

Because people's stages of readiness for change fluctuate, you should assess employees' stages at several points in the program, depending on its length. Some programs have conducted stage assessments at the beginning, at 1 month, and at 3 months (Marcus et al., 1998); however, there is no hard-and-fast rule for how often stage assessment should be done. How frequently you assess participants' behavior and physical activity intentions and what you use to assess their behavior depends on your program goals and ultimately the type of change you need to be able to demonstrate to continue to receive funding or to attract new funding for your program.

Choosing Your Target Audience

One of your first decisions when designing a work site program will be whether to recruit participants reactively (i.e., potential participants come to you) or proactively (i.e., you reach out to potential participants and offer your services). If you decide to start with reactive recruitment strategies (i.e., intervening only with employees who have responded to your program advertisements rather than reaching out to all employees), you will need to have ideas for helping people at various stages of motivational readiness. However, if you proactively recruit participants, you can decide which stage you want your program to target and how you will reach people in that stage.

You may want your first program to focus on those in stage 3, who do some physical activity each week. Your job is to help them become regular exercisers. These people are an easy first target for your program because they are likely to be quite receptive to physical activity messages and events, and they have some ideas about how to get started. To reach them, you could conduct and publicize a fun event, such as an "exercise journey" in which you pick a destination, such as New Orleans during Mardi Gras season; track the time or miles it would take to walk, jog, or swim there; and reward participants when they reach the destination (Glaros, 1997). Such an event promotes the idea that physical activity is important and fun and also encourages your target group members to monitor their progress and reward themselves for reaching a goal. If this event is successful, you can plan how to reach employees at other stages.

Although already active, employees in stage 4, doing enough physical activity, and stage 5, making it a habit, are often the people most interested in physical activity programs offered at work. Special events such as fun runs, fitness assessments, or rewards for physical activity participation can keep them motivated by making their physical activity fun and different from their ordinary routine. Employees in these stages also are likely to be interested in tips for maintaining their activity during difficult times, such as bad weather or illness, and in information about unfamiliar exercise benefits, such as improved immune functioning. These tips and information can be provided in a short monthly newsletter or e-mail message. The fact that these people are already active at the recommended level does not mean that they have little to gain from physical activity promotion. In fact, helping them vary their activities to prevent boredom and relapse is especially important because physical activity behavior is characterized by several starts and stops during a person's lifetime.

Employees in the earliest stages (i.e., stage 1, not thinking about change, and stage 2, thinking about change) are probably the ones that health promoters most want to reach. However, their lack of motivational readiness makes them the hardest to involve in work site physical activity events. Your task is to increase these employees' awareness of the importance of physical activity, reinforce the notion that *anyone* can be physically active, and get them to think about how their current inactivity might affect them and others who are important to them. For this group, motivationally targeted messages that acknowledge their reluctance to become physically active are paramount. For example, ideas for overcoming common barriers may attract these people's attention because they believe that the reasons for being inactive outweigh those for being active. A heading such as *Not Ready to Be Physically Active?* communicates to employees at early stages that the information provided is relevant to them.

Messages aimed at people in the earlier stages and events for employees in the later stages communicate to all employees that physical activity is important to and valued by the employer. This can be crucial in moving people even in the earliest stages toward actually taking part in some physical activity.

Reaching Your Target Audience

A common way to communicate physical activity messages in the workplace is to post them in highly visible places: bulletin boards, the cafeteria, doorways. Sending questions and receiving answers by e-mail is another good option for many work sites. However, people who do not have a current interest in becoming more physically active may not pay much attention to these messages or may quickly dismiss them as irrelevant. Therefore, consider other communication routes that employees routinely use: office mail, paycheck stuffers, voice mail, a brief announcement on the company's intranet. Messages from managers, other employees, the human resources department, employee assistance programs, and union leaders may convince people at the early stages of motivational readiness to at least give physical activity another thought (USDHHS et al., 1999). Using several channels of communication also demonstrates to employees the organization's commitment to physical activity promotion.

Developing Stage-Matched Materials

In addition to written materials that describe the exercise facilities available or how to start an exercise program (e.g., brochures from the AHA such as "Exercise and Your Heart: A Guide to Physical Activity" and "The Walking Handbook"), be sure to also have available materials geared toward people not thinking about activity and those thinking about it but not yet ready to start. Such materials might include a handout on the benefits of regular activity or suggestions for how to deal with common barriers that keep people from exercising. In materials such as these, be sure to applaud the employee for taking the important step of picking up the brochure and reading about exercise. It is helpful to acknowledge in the title or the opening text that the reader may not be thinking of starting a physical activity program now but that the information might be useful if the person starts thinking more seriously about becoming physically active in the future. For example, we have used titles such as "What's in It for Me?" and "Do I Need This?" on materials designed for people in stage 1. This helps readers in the early stages to perceive the materials as relevant to them and thereby increases the likelihood that they will actually read them. Those in the later stages are looking for different information, such as how to prevent injury, how to add variety to their usual physical activity routines, or how to be active during vacations or business trips. Here are some suggested topics for stage-matched written materials. (Copies of stage-matched materials that have been developed and tested in work settings can be ordered by calling 401-793-8081 or e-mailing a request to LSExercise@lifespan.org.)

Topics for Creating Stage-Appropriate Materials

Stage 1: Not thinking about change

- Health benefits of physical activity
- Overcoming common excuses

Stage 2: Thinking about change

- Increasing lifestyle activity
- Considering benefits and barriers
- Setting short- and long-term goals
- Rewarding yourself

Stage 3: Doing some physical activity

- Goal setting
- Developing a walking program

- Tips for enjoying physical activity
- Fitting more activity into a busy schedule

Stage 4: Doing enough physical activity

- Overcoming obstacles
- Preventing boredom
- Gaining social support
- Increasing your confidence in staying active

Stage 5: Making physical activity a habit

- Avoiding injury
- Trying new activities
- Planning ahead for difficult situations
- Rewarding yourself

Focusing on Moderate-Intensity Activity

Many people still adhere to the old adage "no pain, no gain" when it comes to physical activity. This philosophy is particularly unappealing to those who are not motivated to be more physically active. A work site program based on the stages of motivational readiness for change should promote activities that do not take much time or effort, consistent with the philosophy that a little activity is better than none at all. Such activities include taking the stairs rather than the elevator once in a while, parking in the farthest parking space for one day, or taking a walking break. Ask managers to provide their employees with opportunities for physical activity to increase the effectiveness of your program.

Some businesses and employers might be reluctant to promote physical activity because they are concerned about liability issues should an employee become injured as a result of a program they promoted. However, requiring that each employee consult with a physician before beginning a physical activity program puts up another barrier. You can address this concern by letting the employer know that you advocate moderate-intensity activity. Using the Physical Activity Readiness Questionnaire (PAR-Q; see chapter 7) to identify any potential health concerns can allay employers' concerns about this issue.

Planning Events

Ideas for action-oriented events for the workplace, such as walk-a-thons or using a map of the United States to track miles, are readily available (e.g., Glaros, 1997). However, a stage-matched workplace program also should include events that are more personal and informational in nature, such as walking programs, structured classes, and skill-building programs. An example of an event for employees in early stages of motivational readiness is a barriers assessment in which employees take a minute or two to identify their top few reasons for not becoming physically active (they can use the form in figure 7.4); then your program might consist of teaching problem-solving strategies to overcome these barriers. This activity can be done in either an individual or group format.

Another idea is to have employees identify how they might personally benefit from becoming a little more physically active and perhaps sharing this information with a family member or coworker. Finding an article or Web site (e.g., www.americanheart.org) that pertains to physical activity and reading through this information could be a short-term goal for those in the earlier stages. You might also consider having participants share with you the articles or Web sites they found helpful so that you increase your collection of useful materials to distribute to other employees. You can increase employees' awareness of your program by kicking it off with a guest speaker or by giving a gift to each employee, such as a T-shirt, shoelaces, or a water bottle.

Employees in the early stages of motivational readiness may not be interested in becoming more physically active at present, but they might be interested in related issues, such as weight management, smoking cessation, stress reduction, or time management. Addressing these topics can enhance their confidence about physical activity; for example, you can encourage them to use their new time management skills to become active or persuade them that a little physical activity can be helpful in their efforts to manage their weight. These topics also are likely to be relevant to people in stages 3, 4, and 5 and may help them increase or maintain their activity. Thus, programs addressing these topics can be a great use of your time and of management's financial resources.

Adding Incentives for Participation

A review of workplace physical activity interventions found that adding incentives for participation increased programs' effectiveness (Dishman, Oldenburg, O'Neal, & Shephard, 1998). Including several incentives for participation, especially in the beginning, helps employees commit to the program. Financial incentives include additional payment or reimbursement for participation. An employer might collaborate with a local exercise facility to offer a 1-month membership to employees who sign up for the program. Prizes such as T-shirts either for participation or for achievement of physical activity goals also have been used. However, it is important to ensure that the goals are commensurate with the individual employee's baseline motivation level; one employee may hit his goal by reading about physical activity 5 days that week, whereas another employee may need to participate in physical activity 5 days that week to meet her goal. Awards and recognition through trophies, certificates, or announcements in the workplace help create a social norm for physical activity. Listing participants' names in an employee newsletter can also be effective. Release time from work to participate also has been used as an incentive to get employees to participate, although this obviously requires management's support.

The following case example shows how one group of program planners implemented a successful work site physical activity program.

Creating Change in the Workplace

The Jump Start to Health program took place in 11 manufacturing work sites as part of a larger health promotion program that included smoking cessation, nutrition education, and physical activity (Marcus et al., 1998). The physical activity portion was advertised through signs placed around the workplace, and special efforts were made to attract employees who were sedentary and less motivated to become more active. Those who agreed to participate received a $1 Rhode Island lottery ticket as an incentive. Free popcorn and beverages also were offered to employees who filled out the questionnaires used to assess their stages of motivational readiness for physical activity and their physical activity behavior. At most work sites, employees were given time off from work to complete their questionnaires; however, at a few work sites, employees filled out their assessments during break time, lunch, or after work. Assessments were done on laptop computers and took about 15 minutes.

The Jump Start to Health program was designed to test the effectiveness of motivationally tailored print materials based on the stages of change and social cognitive theory versus standard print materials from the American Heart Association (AHA), which are more action oriented. Each employee who agreed to participate was randomly assigned to either the stage-matched intervention or the standard intervention. Participants received print materials at baseline and 1 month later. At baseline, employees assigned to the stage-matched intervention received a manual tailored to their stage of motivational readiness for change. At the 1-month follow-up they received the manual matched to their stage plus the manual for the next stage. The topics included in each of these manuals are provided in chapter 5. Each of the AHA manuals discussed a type of physical activity (e.g., walking, swimming, cycling, aerobic dance, running). Employees assigned to the standard intervention received one of these manuals at baseline. One month later they received the same manual plus one discussing another type of activity.

Change in physical activity behavior was assessed at baseline and then again at 3 months. Analyses of the program's effectiveness revealed that more subjects in the stage-matched group than in the non-stage-matched group progressed in stage of motivational readiness to become more active (37% vs. 27%). The program was particularly effective for those who entered the program in stage 1 (not thinking about change), stage 2 (thinking about change), and stage 3 (doing some physical activity). Stage progression was associated with more minutes spent in physical activity. These results are noteworthy given that work site physical activity programs often attract employees who are already active or more motivated to become active.

CASE EXAMPLE

Stage-Specific Strategies for Work Site Programs

Once you have evaluated employee interest and managerial support for your work site physical activity promotion program, the funds you have available, and the means you are going to use to deliver the program, it is time to put it together. We hope that the following list of stage-specific workplace program strategies will help you generate some ideas for developing a program that will meet the needs of the employees with whom you are working.

STAGE 1

NOT THINKING ABOUT CHANGE

For sedentary employees who are not thinking about physical activity behavior change, an appropriate objective for your program might be to increase their awareness of the benefits of physical activity and the level of activity necessary to obtain these benefits. Here are some strategies for increasing awareness and encouraging these employees to begin to think about the role physical activity could play in their lives.

What are some ways to promote physical activity awareness?

- Kick off your program with a special event such as a guest speaker or by giving T-shirts to every employee (USDHHS et al., 1999).
- Set up informational displays in prominent places such as at the front entrance, in reception areas, by the elevator or stairwell, on bulletin boards, at coffee or snack machines, or in the restrooms, or send information by e-mail (USDHHS et al., 1999).
- Offer an incentive to employees who read or find information on physical activity.
- Distribute print materials targeted toward people who are presently not thinking about becoming more physically active.
- Host a health fair during lunch that includes fitness testing, blood pressure screening, or body fat assessment. Relate how these are affected by physical activity.

What information might get employees to consider physical activity?

- Give a presentation to correct common misconceptions (e.g., you have to exercise vigorously to gain health benefits).
- Present new recommended levels of physical activity and the benefits that can be gained through accumulated moderate-intensity physical activities.
- List lifestyle activities that can help a person achieve health benefits if performed at a moderate intensity (see chapter 6). Notions such as "no pain, no gain" may be leading some to remain at this stage.

What are some strategies for making physical activity personally relevant to these employees?

- Conduct a health fair that offers free physical fitness assessments (USDHHS et al., 1999).

- Do a barriers assessment related to either home or work site physical activity (depending on the goals of your program) and provide suggestions for overcoming barriers.

- Have employees identify how they might personally benefit from becoming physically active.

- Personalize your message to help employees see how it relates to their lives.

- Hold a workshop or seminar on a related topic such as weight loss, time management, stress management, or smoking cessation. Include how physical activity relates to the topic.

- Find out what the employees in your setting desire most and tailor your activities to those goals (weight loss, health benefits, mental health benefits).

What type of special event is particularly relevant for these employees?

- Hold a Top 10 Excuses T-Shirt Contest (Glaros, 1997). Ask employees to submit their best excuse for not exercising. Ask for two excuses—one that is a legitimate problem for them and another that is humorous. Have your employee wellness committee or other staff judge the excuses. Order T-shirts printed with the top 10 excuses.

- Award free T-shirts to the employees who submitted the selected 10 excuses. Offer all entrants support, guidance, or suggestions on how to overcome the legitimate excuses.

- Use the list of entrants as a targeted mailing list for promotion materials.

STAGE 2

THINKING ABOUT CHANGE

For employees in stage 2, one of your objectives might be to increase awareness of the benefits of physical activity and its acceptance in the work community. A second objective would be to move these employees closer to actually trying out the behavior. Here are some ideas for achieving these objectives.

What are some ways to promote physical activity awareness?

- Distribute print materials targeted toward people who are thinking about becoming more physically active.
- Establish a library with educational materials on physical activity (USDHHS et al., 1999).
- Take advantage of New Year's resolutions in January, the start of spring, annual employee physicals, or other dates to post information or hold an event (Glaros, 1997).
- Kick off your program with a special event such as a guest speaker or by giving T-shirts to every employee (USDHHS et al., 1999).
- Set up informational displays in prominent places such as at the front entrance, in reception areas, by the elevator or stairwell, on bulletin boards, at coffee or snack machines, or in the restrooms, or send information by e-mail (USDHHS et al., 1999).
- Offer an incentive to employees who read or find information on physical activity.

What information might get employees to consider physical activity?

- Conduct a health fair that offers free physical fitness assessments (USDHHS et al., 1999).
- Gather and distribute a list of community resources for physical activity (USDHHS et al., 1999).
- Do a barriers assessment related to either home or work site physical activity (depending on the goals of your program) and provide suggestions for overcoming barriers.
- Hold a workshop on developing an activity plan (what, where, when, with whom).

STAGE 2

What strategies might prompt these employees to try some physical activity?

- Provide employees with the opportunity to take a 10-minute walking break during the workday.

- Post cues by the elevator to take the stairs instead of the elevator.

- Have employees set up a "start date" during which time they will complete the goal of 10 minutes of physical activity. Follow up to see how the employees did.

- Suggest that employees walk to a lunch spot that is a couple of blocks away rather than to the in-house cafeteria or the place across the street.

- Give the message that "some activity is better than nothing."

What is an example of a special event that would be appropriate for employees in this stage?

- Host an event called Walk a Mall in My Shoes (Glaros, 1997). Plan a walking route that covers an appropriate distance in a mall. Select stores at appropriate intervals as checkpoints and record some distinctive feature from their window displays such as sales prices, featured items, or unique displays. Create a scavenger hunt with a series of questions that participants must answer during the course of the walk.

- Keep in mind that many of the participants will be sedentary, so be conservative with the distance you expect them to travel. Encourage participants to walk the route in pairs in the order you have indicated.

- Arrange for gift certificates valid in the mall as incentives.

STAGE 3

DOING SOME PHYSICAL ACTIVITY

Employees in stage 3 are likely to be receptive to physical activity promotion in the workplace, given that they are doing some activity but not enough to meet national guidelines. Therefore, your program objective for this group is to encourage them to increase the amount of physical activity they do each week, perhaps by getting more physical activity in at work. To communicate with these employees about your program, you can use various communication channels available at the work site. Here are some ideas to target these employees.

What channels might you use to get your message to these employees?

- Conduct a lunchtime workshop on making time for physical activity or strategies for building in activity routinely throughout the day.
- Start an e-mail program that offers a tip of the day and encourages employees to e-mail reports of their physical activity. Provide encouragement and support through brief e-mailed feedback.
- Post energy expenditure charts.
- Conduct a lunchtime workshop on priority setting for exercise.
- Distribute print materials targeted toward people who are thinking about becoming more physically active.

What strategies might help these employees increase their physical activity?

- Encourage these employees to keep track of how much activity they are doing each week.
- Create a point system for making progress toward a physically active lifestyle. Make points redeemable for meaningful rewards such as donated gifts from local sponsors (USDHHS et al., 1999).
- Post cues by the elevator to take the stairs instead of the elevator.
- Help to set up informal physical activity support networks among the employees (USDHHS et al., 1999).
- Provide exercise prescriptions appropriate to employees' levels of fitness.
- Have employees monitor the minutes they spend sitting and being active during a day. Encourage employees to replace sitting time with activity time (see chapter 6).
- Encourage employees to hold one-on-one meetings while walking.
- Suggest that employees set their computers to beep once an hour as a reminder to take a 2-minute walk.
- Encourage employees to set a realistic goal for increasing the amount of activity they are doing.
- Provide opportunities for employees to practice new physical activity skills in a safe, nonjudgmental environment.

STAGE 3

What is an example of a special event that would be appropriate for employees in this stage?

- Plan an event called Conquering Mount Everest (Glaros, 1997). To prepare for this journey, a few calculations are necessary. The total height of Mount Everest is 29,028 feet (8,848 m). The distance between floors in most office buildings is 13 feet (4 m). One way to set up this journey is to have participants climb 130 feet (40 m) per day (10 floors), 5 days per week. "Trek teams" with four members each would need approximately 11 weeks to complete the event. One person should be designated as the "sherpa" to serve as team organizer and leader. Team members report their climbing success each week to the sherpa, who totals it and reports it to you. Alternatively, you can place a drop box at the bottom of each stairwell with simple forms available for logging progress.

- Encourage your employees to add stair climbing to their daily routines rather than trying to do a week's worth of climbing in one day.

STAGE 4

DOING ENOUGH PHYSICAL ACTIVITY

Employees in stage 4 have recently become active at the level recommended by national guidelines. Your program objective for this group will be to promote continued participation in activity for the long term. To accomplish this, you can use some of the following strategies.

What channels might you use to get your message to these employees?

▪ Distribute print materials targeted toward people who are regularly physically active but only recently so.

▪ Set up a chat room on the intranet for problem solving.

▪ Conduct a lunchtime workshop on preventing boredom with physical activity.

▪ Start an e-mail-based program that offers a tip of the day and encourages employees to e-mail reports of their physical activity. Provide encouragement and support through brief e-mailed feedback.

What strategies might help these employees keep up their physical activity?

▪ Teach skills in alternative activities (in-line skating, tennis, kickboxing, Tae Bo).

▪ Encourage employees to come up with a plan for maintaining or resuming physical activity during times when work or life is especially hectic.

▪ Sponsor an event that includes family and friends.

▪ Post mile markers on work site grounds or measure the distance of inside routes (USDHHS et al., 1999).

▪ Negotiate deals for employees to use local exercise facilities.

▪ Give employees points for time spent being physically active each week and make points redeemable for small gift items such as exercise clothing, movie tickets, or passes to local exercise facilities or dances (USDHHS et al., 1999).

What further activities would be appropriate for employees in this stage?

▪ Encourage support groups (Glaros, 1997). Use surveys and focus groups to establish what these employees need. Create a mailing list of targeted employees and send them supportive messages.

▪ Publicize your physical activity intervention group and establish an initial meeting time, date, and place. Arrange for a content expert to be present at the initial meeting (who may also be available at future meetings on an as-needed basis). At the meeting, introduce your expert, determine the goals of the group, and share your own ideas for the group.

▪ Identify potential group leaders who can assist in communications and logistics. Establish a proposed meeting schedule and use your connections to reserve rooms and obtain management permission if needed.

▪ Attend occasional meetings yourself to keep in touch with employees' activities and status.

STAGE 5

MAKING PHYSICAL ACTIVITY A HABIT

Employees in stage 5 are familiar with physical activity because they have been regularly active for at least 6 months. Your program objective will be to help them keep active by anticipating lapses, planning for situations that jeopardize their activity, and keeping them motivated over the long term. Here are some suggestions for achieving these goals.

What strategies might help these employees prevent setbacks in their physical activity?

- Distribute print materials targeted toward people who are active and have been so for at least 6 months.
- Sponsor a charity walk or run.
- Give away step counters, self-monitoring booklets, or magnets with a self-monitoring form to encourage continued goal setting (see chapter 6).
- Ask these employees to sponsor a friend, family member, or coworker who is trying to get started with physical activity.
- Give a workshop on injury prevention.
- Teach skills in alternative activities to prevent boredom.

What is an example of a special event that would be appropriate for employees in this stage?

- National Jogging Day, which takes place in October, is an opportunity to either end the primary running season, or, especially in northern regions, prepare participants for, and encourage participants to continue, running through the difficult winter months (Glaros, 1997).
- Organize a 5K fun walk or run. Consider including family members for team events (for example, father and son) (Glaros, 1997).
- Begin a walking or running program with a destination-based or distance goal that culminates on either Thanksgiving or New Year's Day (Glaros, 1997).
- If your workplace is located in an area where the climate changes, host a seminar on performing physical activity in cold weather featuring both training methods and specialized clothing.
- Use the seminar to introduce running to interested nonrunners.
- Organize a series of events featuring motorized treadmills as an alternative to outdoor winter walking or running.
- Promote active participation in your walking club, especially for new members.
- Develop a list of locations, such as local colleges and community sport facilities, that are suitable for indoor physical activity during the winter months. If possible, provide maps of locations (Glaros, 1997).

Conclusion

Because many Americans work outside the home, work site physical activity programs have the potential to reach a lot of people. Traditional work site programs have tended to attract only employees most motivated to be physically active. However, a stage-matched approach, as described in this chapter, can attract and retain greater numbers of employees than traditional programs can. We hope that this chapter has provided some useful ideas for developing and implementing a physical activity program to meet the needs of all employees at your work site.

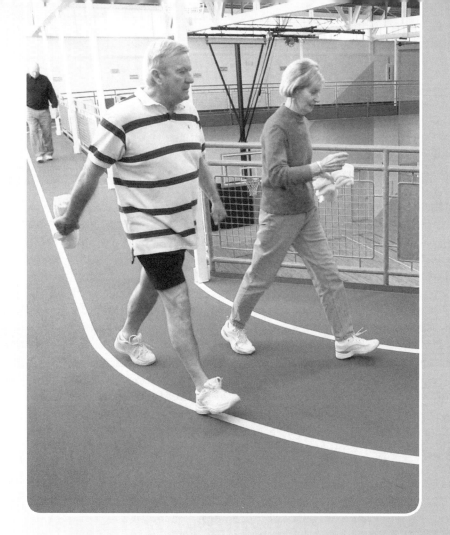

Using the Stages Model in Community Programs

By designing and implementing a community-based physical activity program, you can make an impact on the public health of your community, but developing a program to meet the needs of an entire community can be a daunting task. The people within any given community are sure to differ significantly, so whom should you target? What type of program can help these people the most? Such a large-scale project may also be expensive. However, community programs have the potential to reach a great number of underactive people through various channels, such as the mass media, print materials, and community leaders, and through organized events such as fun runs and health fairs. You can also reach a larger number of people in the community at a low cost per person by taking advantage of technologies such as the telephone, interactive computer systems, and the Internet (Marcus, Owen, Forsyth, Cavill, & Fridinger, 1998; Marcus et al., 2007; Marshall, Owen, & Bauman, 2004).

Community campaigns to improve cardiovascular health that have included physical activity have been around for over three decades. Programs such as the Stanford Five-City Project (Young, Haskel, Taylor, & Fortmann, 1996) and the Minnesota Heart Health Program (Luepker, Murray, Jacobs, & Mittelmark, 1994) have targeted several cardiovascular risk factors, including high blood pressure, poor diet, and tobacco use, while promoting physical activity. In the past, community-based projects tended to use a one-size-fits-all approach, in which a general message promoting physical activity was given to all people, regardless of their level of motivational readiness for taking up physical activity. Although programs such as these helped increase awareness of the benefits of physical activity, they were less effective at increasing physical activity behavior (Marcus, Owen, et al., 1998).

We have since learned that it is important to divide the population into subgroups (i.e., target audiences) and customize programs for each of these segments to better meet the needs of people within a community. Studies that have divided populations by motivational stage of readiness and then delivered stage-targeted messages have proven to be more successful than traditional approaches for getting people to change their behavior (Marcus, Bock, et al., 1998; Marcus, Emmons et al., 1998; Will, Farris, Sander, Stockmyer & Finklestein, 2004). Chapter 5 provides a more detailed description of some of these programs, such as Jump Start, Project STRIDE, and Step Into Motion.

In this chapter we discuss how you can use the stages of motivational readiness to design a physical activity program for the people in your community and strategies that might be effective for these people. You can also refer to *Promoting Physical Activity: A Guide for Community Action* (USDHHS et al., 1999), which is an excellent resource for designing and implementing a community program. To begin, we discuss reasons to use the stages of motivational readiness to build your program.

Assessing the Community's Readiness for Change

Traditionally, the stages of motivational readiness for change model is used to describe behavior change at the individual level (USDHHS et al., 1999). However, some have also applied it to entire communities to describe how ready a given community is to make physical activity a priority for its residents (Abrams, 1991; McLeroy, Bibeau, Steckler, & Glanz, 1998; USDHHS et al., 1999). Researchers and health promoters alike have noted that environmental factors are important considerations for individual behavior change (Heath et al., 2006; Humpel, Owen, & Leslie, 2002; Kahn et al., 2002). For example, sidewalks and bike and walking paths enhance the likelihood of individual behavior change. Institutional factors also affect individual change, such as an employer who does not give employees release time for physical activity. The stages of physical activity readiness at a community level are also influenced by societal factors, such as support from community officials. As illustrated in figure 10.1, environmental, social, and institutional factors influence each other and are all important considerations in a community's readiness for change. Here are other specific examples of how the stages of change can be interpreted at a community level (USDHHS et al., 1999, p. 62):

- A work site that is considering a change in employee health benefits to include physical activity incentives might be in stage 2, thinking about change.
- A work site whose administration is already taking the appropriate steps to institutionalize a cost-effective physical activity program might be in stage 5, making activity a habit.
- A school district that is piloting a model physical activity program in one of its schools may be in stage 3, doing some physical activity, before adopting the program district wide.
- A community in the construction phase of converting old railroad lines into pedestrian and bicycle pathways has demonstrated that the community is in stage 4, or the action phase.

Determining the stage of motivational readiness of a community helps you learn the barriers to change at the community level (e.g., unsafe neighborhoods for walking, few activity-related events, lack of support from community officials) and the potential community supports for physical activity (e.g., health care providers willing to counsel their patients on physical activity, work site wellness groups already in place). The community's motivational readiness for physical activity promotion can be determined in various ways. You might

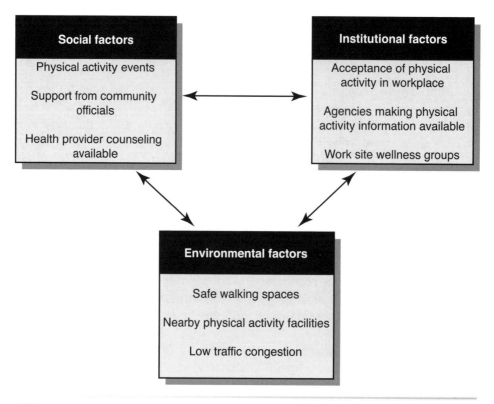

FIGURE 10.1   The influence of social, institutional, and environmental factors on community readiness for change.

examine the community's physical environment, or you might interview several community members of different ages, social classes, and so forth, to see whether they believe community support is in place for them to become or stay physically active (e.g., safe walking areas, acceptance of physical activity in the workplace, nearby community exercise facilities). You also should determine the community's commitment to physical activity–related goals or practices. For example, are agencies willing to make physical activity information available? Are activity-related events taking place?

Your stage assessment should include the community's status on physical activity–promoting actions, its intention to move toward them, and the steps it has taken or the plan it has in place for implementing them (USDHHS et al., 1999). You will also need to assess the community's ability to achieve specific behavioral goals related to physical activity (USDHHS et al., 1999). Such behavioral goals might include the following actions in these areas:

■ **Social networks.** Develop community walking groups. Foster collaborations among local health agencies. Encourage partnerships between businesses and exercise facilities. Generate a hotline to offer ideas, information, and encouragement to members of the community.

- **Environment.** Raise funds for more biking and walking paths. Build housing developments near exercise facilities. Promote public transportation. Install better lighting for sidewalks.

- **Community norms.** Encourage biking with helmets as a way to travel to work. Publicize the need for child care in fitness facilities. Have community leaders deliver physical activity messages.

- **Policies and legislation.** Lobby for tax cuts for work sites that promote physical activity for their employees. Pass zoning laws for green space.

Once you have determined the community's stage of motivational readiness for various program ideas that you have in mind, you can begin to think about how to meet the needs of individuals within the community.

Reaching Individuals Within a Community

A goal of influencing everyone in a given community is unrealistic. Programs that try to do so end up serving no one very well. As mentioned earlier, general programs do not account for individual differences that affect physical activity adoption. A more appropriate goal for a community physical activity program is to reach a majority of people within the community.

To make a program work for a large number of people, you must assess the needs of the people you are trying to reach (USDHHS et al., 1999). You can determine the stages of most people in the community, or you can choose a target audience and then determine the stages of the people within it. Before designing your program, find out what the people in your target audience think about physical activity, why they might want to become more active, what has been holding them back, where they go to get their information, and possible sources of support. You can then customize your message to meet their needs.

This approach of designing your program around the needs of your target audience is based on business marketing principles called social marketing (Kotler & Zaltman, 1971). Social marketing is an approach in which the marketer listens to what consumers believe is best for them and formulates the solution to suit consumers' perceptions rather than trying to tell consumers what is best for them. Consumers' perceptions can be obtained through focus groups and personal interviews with representative people from the selected audience. The 12 CDC-funded WISEWOMAN projects conducted across the United States have demonstrated that this social marketing approach can yield positive results, even for populations that are typically difficult to reach.

CASE EXAMPLE

Creating Change Within the Community

The WISEWOMAN (Well-Integrated Screening and Evaluation for Women Across the Nation) projects were developed by the CDC to provide early screening and promote healthy lifestyles in middle-aged, financially disadvantaged women across the country (Will, Farris, Sanders, Stockmyer, & Finklestein, 2004). Under-insured and uninsured women aged 50 to 64 participating in the National Breast and Cervical Cancer Early Detection Program (NBCCEDP) were recruited to also participate in the WISEWOMAN project for the prevention of cardiovascular disease through their NBCCEDP clinic sites. Half of the clinic sites provided a minimum intervention (MI) of screening, referral, and follow-up as needed. The clinic sites providing the enhanced intervention (EI) also included interventions based on social cognitive theory and the socioecological model to encourage healthy eating, smoking cessation, and moderate-intensity physical activity. The specific physical activity intervention strategies employed varied across the states. Participants in the EI reported increased levels of moderate-to-vigorous physical activity at 12-month follow-up compared to participants in the MI (Jacobs et al., 2004; Staten et al., 2004; Stoddard, Palombo, Troped, Sorensen, & Will, 2004).

Looking more specifically at the Massachusetts program, the EI included tailoring, self-monitoring, readiness for change, self-efficacy, shaping, social support, and overcoming barriers (Stoddard et al., 2004). Participants received individual physical activity assessments, one-on-one physical activity counseling based on the Physician Assisted Counseling and Evaluation (PACE) program (Calfas et al., 2002), walking groups, lists of community resources for physical activity, and peer social support (Stoddard et al., 2004). Three-fourths of the intervention activities for the various health behaviors included a physical activity component to provide participants with repeated opportunities to build physical activity skills. Furthermore, women participating in the EI arm of the study helped to select and design the physical activity components in which they were going to participate. Social interaction and social support were encouraged in these activities. As a result, 96% of the participants reported being very satisfied with the physical activity component of the program, and social support was found to be associated with increased physical activity. The authors of the Massachusetts study concluded that designing interventions that are culturally and age appropriate, providing repeated exposure to physical activity opportunities, and increasing social support appear to be promising strategies for effective physical activity programs for underserved women.

Developing Stage-Matched Messages

Targeting and tailoring are two social marketing strategies that can be very useful for communicating physical activity messages (figure 10.2). Target-

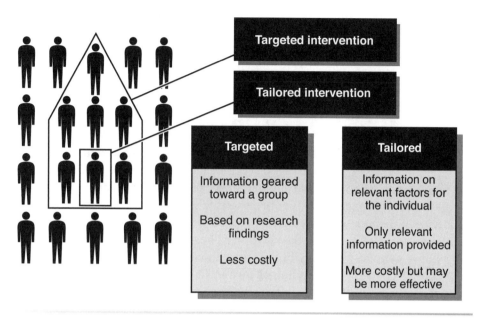

FIGURE 10.2 Targeted versus tailored approaches to physical activity promotion.

ing a program involves defining groups within the population along some characteristic, such as stage of motivational readiness, and then delivering a program suited to this characteristic. A targeted approach assumes that the members of a defined group are similar enough for one message to effectively communicate to all members of the group. Targeting by stage of motivational readiness and then delivering stage-matched printed materials about physical activity have been shown to effectively increase physical activity behavior (Marcus et al., 1992; Marcus, Emmons, et al., 1998). Chapter 5 provides more detailed descriptions of these programs, such as Imagine Action and Jump Start: A Community-Based Study.

A tailored program is customized to each member according to his or her stage of motivational readiness. Personally relevant messages are created based on each person's answers to questions about factors such as self-efficacy, use of relevant cognitive and behavioral strategies, and outcome expectations (Marcus, Nigg, Riebe, & Forsyth, 2000). Although the tailored approach requires more testing, we believe that providing people with personally relevant messages will increase the likelihood that they read and process the messages. This in turn should increase the likelihood that they use the information to change their behavior.

Although providing individually tailored, stage-matched messages about physical activity sounds ideal, doing so is more expensive and labor intensive than delivering a single targeted message. You need to weigh the costs and benefits when deciding between a targeted and tailored approach. In some cases, technologies such as computers and the Internet can be cost effective in individually tailoring physical activity messages. Moreover, technologies such as these allow us to move beyond reliance on face-to-face counseling to affordable, individually tailored counseling (see chapter 5 for a description of programs that used computer-generated tailored messages, such as Jump Start: A Community-Based Study [Marcus, Bock, et al., 1998] and Project STRIDE [Marcus, Napolitano, et al., 2007]).

Using a Media-Based Approach to Reach Your Target Audience

Reviews of published physical activity studies reveal that interventions using a media-based approach to deliver programs (e.g., print mailings, telecommunications) can be more effective than programs delivered face to face (Dishman & Buckworth, 1996). Media-based approaches may be more effective because they allow people more flexibility and choice in how they implement their physical activity programs, whereas face-to-face programs usually entail some type of physical activity done in the presence of the counselor. Moreover, most households can be reached by mail, telephone, or the Internet.

Print

Print-based, stage-targeted physical activity programs delivered to sedentary adults by mail have been found to help them become more active (e.g., Cardinal & Sachs, 1996; Marcus et al., 1992), as have print-based, tailored, self-help physical activity programs (Marcus, Bock, et al., 1998). Participants can be mailed the stages of change questionnaire (questionnaire 2.1 in appendix A) along with other relevant measures, such as the processes of change, self-efficacy, and decisional balance questionnaires (questionnaires 4.1, 4.2, and 4.4 in appendix A). They can then receive personally relevant printed materials within a day or two of mailing their questionnaires.

Telephone

The telephone is another avenue for reaching large numbers of people within a community, given that most Americans have telephones in their homes. Moreover, physical activity counseling by telephone helps sedentary people become more active. For example, a study in which health educators with bachelor's degrees counseled sedentary older adults by telephone about home-based physical activity found that telephone counseling led to better adherence to moderate- and vigorous-intensity physical activity programs than a structured exercise class did (King, Haskell, Taylor, Kraemer, & DeBusk, 1991; King, Taylor, Haskell, & DeBusk, 1988).

Another study compared the effectiveness of physical activity counseling provided via telephone by a health educator and that provided via computer that participants accessed by telephone (King et al., 2002; King et al., 2007). In the computer-based program, participants used the touch pads on their telephones to enter their weekly minutes of activity or their intentions to become active, their activity goals for the upcoming week, and whether they wanted to hear information on relevant topics regarding physical activity. The computer system stored their data and delivered recorded voice messages that were appropriate for their stages of motivational readiness. Telephone programs such as these have the advantage of providing on-the-spot support and feedback (Marcus et al., 2000), and they have been shown to be effective in previous studies (Pinto et al., 2000). They also can be used proactively to call people rather than waiting for people to call in to the system. Moreover, people can also call in for physical activity counseling when they feel the need, regardless of the time of day or the day of the week (Marcus et al., 2000). Receiving physical activity counseling at any time when needed is usually not an option when a real person delivers the counseling.

Internet

Internet use has increased dramatically; 73% of American adults had access as of 2005 (Madden, 2006; Madden & Rainie, 2003). Eight out of 10 Internet users have looked online for health information (Fox, 2006; Rees, 2005), and 13% seek information specifically about fitness and nutrition (Fox, 2006). Because a significant number of Internet users currently seek health information online, this number is likely to increase as health and fitness Web sites increase in number, especially those that provide information tailored to the user (e.g., www.shapeup.org). There are other physical activity Web sites listed in appendix B.

Programs such as Step Into Motion (Marcus, Lewis et al., 2007; see chapter 5 for a more detailed description), in which the participants answered stages of change questions on a Web site and then were given stage-relevant messages and links to other relevant stage-appropriate material, found that this delivery mode helped sedentary adults become more active at 6-month and 12-month follow-ups.

Using the World Wide Web to deliver a physical activity program allows participants to get the information in which they are interested and also teaches them to gather information for themselves. E-mail and online chat boards are avenues for providing support and encouragement from program leaders and other program participants, again, at any time of the day or night. Whenever a person is experiencing a barrier or dealing with a lapse, help is available. Technologies such as the Internet and computerized telephone systems are not only more cost-effective than face-to-face programs, but they also provide the community with better access to physical activity advice.

Working With Community Leaders to Reach Your Target Audience

Another promising method for delivering community physical activity programs is through the people who have the greatest influence over the groups of people you are trying to reach (King, 1998). These influential people might include physicians, reporters, journalists, and teachers. For example, you can develop a credit-granting continuing education course about physical activity promotion to train physicians, nurses, psychologists, and other health professionals to deliver stage-matched physical activity counseling to their patients (King, 1998). Similarly, you can offer training to physical education instructors in promoting lifestyle activity by encouraging them to use relevant cognitive and behavioral strategies with their students (King, 1998). Politicians, members of the clergy, and other community leaders also influence public opinion and can be helpful by endorsing your program to the community or at least to their constituents in the community you are targeting.

Stage-Specific Strategies for Community Physical Activity Programs

We created the following list of intervention strategies to help you design your own community program. As we have tried to stress in this and other chapters, no one program works for everyone, so we do not provide a step-by-step program development guide. Rather, we hope you pick some of the following strategies plus generate some of your own ideas so that you create a program that addresses the needs of your target audience, your community's stage of change, any time constraints you may be working under, and your financial resources.

STAGE 1

NOT THINKING ABOUT CHANGE

For this segment of the population, your goal is to help increase awareness about the (a) benefits of physical activity, (b) support for it in the local community, and (c) acceptance of physical activity by other community members. Here are some strategies for increasing awareness and encouraging people to begin to think about the role physical activity could play in their lives.

What communication channels might you use to reach people not considering becoming active?

- Distribute print materials targeted toward people who are presently not thinking about becoming more physically active.
- Work with the media to gain visibility for your messages. You might achieve this by doing the following (USDHHS et al., 1999):

STAGE 1

- Invite newspaper reporters to visible or newsworthy events.
- Work with reporters in writing feature stories.
- Provide timely news releases or newspaper articles.
- Participate as a guest on radio or television talk shows.
- Purchase radio, television, or cable advertising time.

∎ Display key messages and your program logo in storefront windows, on community bulletin boards, on billboard signs, and on banners strung across the main street or at major community locations (USDHHS et al., 1999).

∎ Design bumper stickers with physical activity and health promotion messages (USDHHS et al., 1999).

∎ Ask utility companies, banks, physicians, and others to place promotional and educational information in their monthly billings. Ask to place promotional and educational materials in waiting rooms of hospitals and health maintenance organizations, private physicians' offices, clinics, mental health centers, and senior citizen centers (USDHHS et al., 1999).

What types of information are most relevant to people in this earliest stage?

∎ Host health fairs that include exercise testing, blood pressure screenings, or body fat composition assessments. Relate how these are affected by physical activity.

∎ Emphasize the short-term benefits of being active (e.g., feeling invigorated, sleeping better, reducing stress, feeling better about oneself) rather than the long-term benefits that these people might believe are unobtainable.

∎ Dispel misconceptions about physical activity (e.g., "No pain, no gain," overestimated risk of injuries such as heart attack).

∎ Increase awareness of what they might miss by choosing not to be active (e.g., enjoyment from being active, better self-esteem).

What are some other strategies that might move these people closer to considering change?

∎ Help people to visualize success—to visualize a happy, healthy, and active lifestyle.

∎ Encourage these people to read or think about how physical activity might benefit them. For this group, it is better to focus on the benefits of physical activity and not to dwell on the risks of a sedentary lifestyle.

∎ Link the benefits of a physically active lifestyle to people's highest priorities and values in life (e.g., relationship with family, personal faith, health, or happiness).

∎ Encourage these people to see how their sedentary behavior affects them personally and others in their lives (e.g., a sedentary parent models an unhealthy lifestyle to her children).

(continued) ▷

STAGE 1

STAGE 1

STAGE 1 *(continued)*

How might you show community support for physical activity?

■ Encourage health care providers to advise their patients on how they might benefit from physical activity.

■ Choose a spokesperson that the target audience trusts, respects, believes, or can identify with to help increase awareness. Identify role models within the community. Recruit local people to endorse your program (USDHHS et al., 1999).

■ Conduct targeted informational campaigns and sessions (USDHHS et al., 1999) such as the following:

  • Lunch-'n'-learn or community lectures
  • Workshops, seminars, or adult education classes
  • Youth group programs
  • One-on-one counseling or instruction
  • Guest talk-show appearances on television and radio
  • Columns or featured articles in the newspaper

■ Give informative presentations at work sites, in schools, and to community organizations such as Rotary Clubs, Business and Professional Women, or the American Association of Retired Persons (USDHHS et al., 1999).

STAGE 2

THINKING ABOUT CHANGE

For this segment of the community, one of your goals is to increase awareness of the benefits of physical activity, community support, and the social norms for this behavior. Another goal is to move these people closer to actually trying out the behavior. Here are some ideas for achieving these goals.

What communication channels might you use?

- Distribute print materials targeted toward people who are thinking about becoming more physically active or include health and physical activity tips in general publications (USDHHS et al., 1999).
- Increase awareness by working with the media to gain visibility for your messages (USDHHS et al., 1999):
  - Invite newspaper reporters to visible or newsworthy events.
  - Work with reporters in writing feature stories.
  - Provide timely news releases or newspaper articles.
  - Participate as a guest on radio or television talk shows.
  - Purchase radio, television, or cable advertising time.
- Display key messages and your program logo in storefront windows, on community bulletin boards, on billboard signs, and on banners strung across the main street or at major community locations (USDHHS et al., 1999).
- Design bumper stickers with physical activity and health promotion messages.
- Ask utility companies, banks, physicians, and others to place promotional and educational information in their monthly billings. Ask to place promotional and educational materials in waiting rooms of hospitals and health maintenance organizations, private physicians' offices, clinics, mental health centers, and senior citizen centers (USDHHS et al., 1999).
- Make health videos available at video stores and libraries.
- Set up a Web site with links to relevant stage-appropriate physical activity and health sites.

What types of information are most relevant to people who are considering becoming more active?

- Provide basic information about what is needed to achieve a physically active lifestyle such as selecting the appropriate shoes or clothing (USDHHS et al., 1999).
- Describe a variety of activities available to most people that can be done alone or with family and friends.
- Suggest ways to build in some activity into one's daily routine (e.g., taking the stairs at work).
- Dispel misconceptions about physical activity (e.g., "No pain, no gain," overestimated risk of injury such as heart attack).

(continued) ▷

STAGE 2

STAGE 2 *(continued)*

What are some other strategies that might move these people closer to trying some physical activity?

■ Provide messages that link physical activity to values or issues relevant to your target audience.

■ Help them weigh the pros and cons of a physically active lifestyle. Focus on the costs of changing (effort, energy, and the things they must give up to overcome a sedentary lifestyle) and how they might deal with them.

■ Encourage them to start off slowly (e.g., a 5- or 10-minute walk) and build gradually (add 5 minutes per day per week) and explain how to reward themselves when they achieve their goals.

■ Give out self-assessment questionnaires such as the Physical Activity Readiness Questionnaire (PAR-Q, found in chapter 7) and the decisional balance questionnaire (questionnaire 4.4 in appendix A).

■ Help people to visualize success—to visualize a happy, healthy, and active lifestyle.

How might you show community support for trying some physical activity?

■ Host health fairs that include exercise testing, blood pressure screenings, or body fat composition assessments. Relate how these are affected by physical activity.

■ Choose a spokesperson that the target audience trusts, respects, believes, or can identify with. Identify role models within the community. Recruit local people to endorse your program (USDHHS et al., 1999).

■ Encourage health care providers to advise these patients on how they might benefit from physical activity and some steps they could take to begin a physically active lifestyle.

■ Conduct targeted informational campaigns and sessions (USDHHS et al., 1999) such as the following:

• Lunch-'n'-learn or community lectures
• Workshops, seminars, or adult education classes
• Youth group programs
• One-on-one counseling or instruction
• Guest talk-show appearances on television and radio
• Columns or featured articles in the newspaper

■ Give informative presentations at work sites, in schools, and to community organizations such as Rotary Clubs, Business and Professional Women, or the American Association of Retired Persons (USDHHS et al., 1999).

■ Set up physical activity hotlines that people can call with questions about physical activity (USDHHS et al., 1999).

STAGE 3

DOING SOME PHYSICAL ACTIVITY

People in this stage are likely to be receptive to physical activity messages because they are doing some activity but not enough to meet national guidelines. Therefore, your goal for this group is to encourage them to increase the amount of physical activity they do each week. To accomplish this goal, you might choose to do some of the following.

What communication channels might you use to reach these people?

- Distribute print materials targeted toward people who want to become more physically active.
- Develop or make available self-instructional materials, such as DVD instruction, CDs, computer-based instruction, how-to guides, manuals, and kits (USDHHS et al., 1999).
- Provide formal and informal activity-oriented instructional programs, such as workshops, classes, seminars, demonstrations, lessons, and lectures (USDHHS et al., 1999).
- Sponsor "meet the expert" events so community members can learn directly from those who have mastered various skills (USDHHS et al., 1999).
- Set up hotlines people can call with questions about physical activity (USDHHS et al., 1999).
- Set up a Web site with links to relevant physical activity and health sites.

What types of information are most relevant to people who need to increase their level of physical activity?

- Discuss how to develop a plan for regular activity.
- Provide ideas for making activity more fun.
- Teach methods of self-monitoring to keep track of progress.
- Discuss barriers to physical activity and ways to overcome them.
- Suggest ways people might restructure their environments to increase the possibility that they will be active (e.g., move exercise equipment where they will see it rather than hiding it in the basement; keep walking shoes at work or by the door at home).
- Discuss ways to use exercise or sports equipment properly and safely.
- Describe stretching, warm-up, and cool-down techniques.

(continued) ▶

STAGE 3 *(continued)*

What are some other strategies that might move these people closer to meeting national guidelines for regular activity?

- Host health and fitness fairs that include exercise testing to demonstrate that each person needs more physical activity (USDHHS et al., 1999).
- Emphasize small, specific, and realistic goals.
- Encourage the use of self-rewards for meeting goals.
- Encourage people to make use of social support networks such as walking clubs or friends or coworkers who exercise during lunch breaks.
- Suggest exercising while sitting in a chair, standing, or watching television.
- Start a walking or jogging program.

How might you show community support for increasing physical activity?

- Develop a community resource list so that people will know where to find courses or opportunities to develop skills.
- Appeal to the community's competitive spirit with contests, prizes, incentives, publicity, recognition, rewards, and fun promotional items. Establish competitive programs among individuals, neighborhoods, churches, organizations, or businesses. Incentives might include discounts at recreational facilities, fitness club memberships, sports or exercise equipment or apparel, a free lunch, a book, a T-shirt, a pair of walking shoes, public recognition, and community awards (USDHHS et al., 1999).
- Encourage health care providers to advise their patients to increase their levels of physical activity and to take advantage of the many community resources you can identify.
- Provide opportunities to try various types of physical activity for just one day or one event (USDHHS et al., 1999):
  - Community walking events
  - Using stairs instead of elevators for 1 day or 1 week
  - Bicycle-to-work day or other bicycling events
  - Periodic fun runs
  - Lunchtime walking groups at local businesses, schools, or shopping malls
  - Trial memberships and guest passes to use recreational facilities
- For groups of various ages or levels of experience, work with physical education instructors, physical therapists, or exercise physiologists to design appropriate and quality instructional programs.

STAGE 4

DOING ENOUGH PHYSICAL ACTIVITY

These people have recently become active at the level recommended by national guidelines. Your goal is to foster continued participation in physical activity and to bolster continued community support for activity. To accomplish this, you can do some of the following.

What communication channels might you use to reach regularly active people?

■ Distribute print materials targeted toward people who are physically active at the level recommended by national guidelines but at risk for relapse.

■ Set up telephone hotlines people can call with questions about physical activity (USDHHS et al., 1999).

■ Develop a community resource list so that people will know where to find courses or opportunities to develop new skills.

■ Sponsor "meet the expert" events so that community members can learn directly from those who have mastered various skills (USDHHS et al., 1999).

■ Set up a Web site with links to relevant physical activity and health sites.

What types of information are most relevant to people who are regularly active?

■ Provide a list of activities that will reduce the risk of injury and boredom and encourage people to try different activities.

■ Describe stretching, warm-up, and cool-down techniques.

■ Suggest ways to restructure their environment (e.g., move exercise equipment where they will see it rather than hiding it in the basement; keep walking shoes at work or by the door at home) to increase the possibility that they will choose an active pursuit rather than a sedentary one.

■ Instruct on how to avoid the risk of injury from exercise.

■ Teach self-monitoring methods for keeping track of progress.

What are some other strategies to help these people stay active?

■ Encourage the use of social support networks such as walking clubs or friends or coworkers who exercise during lunch breaks.

■ Instruct on how to anticipate lapses and accept them as a normal part of the change process so that the occasional lapse is not viewed as a failure.

■ Help identify situations that are more likely to lead to a lapse and develop a plan for keeping active in these situations.

(continued) ▶

STAGE 4 *(continued)*

- Encourage these people to build in rewards to maintain motivation. These can be tangible, such as a new pair of walking shoes, or intangible, such as making a mental note of achieving a goal.
- Help these people develop long-term goals (e.g., participating in a 5-mile [8K] fun walk in a few months) and short-term goals to help reach their long-term goals (e.g., increasing the distance walked by half a mile [0.8 km] per week).

How might you show community support for staying physically active at nationally recommended levels?

- Appeal to the community's competitive spirit with contests, prizes, incentives, publicity, recognition, rewards, and fun promotional items. Establish competitive programs among individuals, neighborhoods, churches, organizations, or businesses. Incentives might include discounts at recreational facilities, fitness club memberships, sports or exercise equipment or apparel, a free lunch, a book, a T-shirt, a pair of walking shoes, public recognition, and community awards (USDHHS et al., 1999).
- Encourage health care providers to ask their patients about physical activity and tell their patients about community resources for physical activity.
- Provide opportunities to try different types of physical activity for just one day or one event (USDHHS et al., 1999):
  - Community walking events
  - Using stairs instead of elevators for 1 day or 1 week
  - Bicycle-to-work day or other bicycling events
  - Periodic fun runs
  - Lunchtime walking groups at local businesses, schools, or shopping malls
  - Trial memberships and guest passes to use recreational facilities

STAGE 5

MAKING PHYSICAL ACTIVITY A HABIT

People in this group are familiar with physical activity because they have been regularly active for at least 6 months. Your goal is to help them keep active by anticipating lapses, planning for situations that jeopardize their activity, and keeping them motivated over the long term. Here are some suggestions for achieving these goals.

What communication channels might you use to reach regularly active people?

- Distribute print materials targeted toward people who are active and have been for at least 6 months.
- Set up telephone hotlines that people can call with questions about physical activity or activity-related injuries (USDHHS et al., 1999).
- Develop a community resource list so that people will know where to find courses or opportunities to develop new activity skills.
- Sponsor "meet the expert" events so community members can learn directly from those who have mastered various skills that may be new to these people (USDHHS et al., 1999).

What types of information are most relevant to people in this stage?

- Teach how to anticipate lapses and accept them as a normal part of the change process so that the occasional lapse is not viewed as a failure.
- Help people identify situations likely to lead to lapses and encourage them to develop plans for keeping active in these situations.
- Remind regularly active people to build in rewards to maintain motivation. These can be tangible, such as a new pair of walking shoes, or intangible, such as making a mental note of achieving a goal.
- Provide a list of activities that will reduce the risk of injury and boredom and encourage them to try different activities.

What are some other strategies to help these people stay active?

- Encourage the use of social support networks such as walking clubs or friends or coworkers who exercise during lunch breaks.
- Help people recognize and appreciate their personal responsibility for maintaining change.
- Suggest how these people might serve as role models for others.

(continued) ▶

STAGE 5 *(continued)*

How might you show community support for the maintenance of regular physical activity?

▪ Appeal to the community's competitive spirit with contests, prizes, incentives, publicity, recognition, rewards, and fun promotional items. Establish competitive programs among individuals, neighborhoods, churches, organizations, or businesses. Incentives might include discounts at recreational facilities, fitness club memberships, sports or exercise equipment or apparel, a free lunch, a book, a T-shirt, a pair of walking shoes, public recognition, and community awards (USDHHS et al., 1999).

▪ Encourage health care providers to ask their patients about physical activity and counsel them on relapse prevention.

▪ Provide opportunities to try different types of physical activity for just one day or one event (USDHHS et al., 1999):
   • Community walking events
   • Using stairs instead of elevators for 1 day or 1 week
   • Bicycle-to-work day or other bicycling events
   • Periodic fun runs
   • Lunchtime walking groups at local businesses, schools, or shopping malls
   • Trial memberships and guest passes to use recreational facilities

Conclusion

Once you have determined whom you want to target in your community program, what that group's needs and perceptions about physical activity are, the types of messages you want to deliver, and the means by which you will deliver your program, it is time to put your program together. The strategies you select should be based on the scale of your project and the funds available. The Stage-Specific Strategies section offers some suggestions for print materials, media coverage, and community events based on your target audience's motivational readiness for changing their physical activity behavior. You can use these and your own ideas to improve physical activity participation in your community.

APPENDIX A

QUESTIONNAIRES

This book's focus was to translate theories and concepts from behavioral science research into a handbook useful for health professionals who are involved in planning, developing, implementing, or evaluating physical activity programs. Questionnaires can be a valuable tool for those health professionals who are undertaking such roles. In the following pages, please find the questionnaires referenced throughout the book. Copy them and use them to help you develop effective physical activity interventions. (For more detailed information about scoring these questionnaires, please see chapter 4.)

QUESTIONNAIRE 2.1 Physical Activity Stages of Change

For each of the following questions, please circle Yes or No. Please be sure to read the questions carefully.

Physical activity or exercise includes activities such as walking briskly, jogging, bicycling, swimming, or any other activity in which the exertion is at least as intense as these activities.

	No	Yes
1. I am currently physically active.	0	1
2. I intend to become more physically active in the next 6 months.	0	1

For activity to be *regular*, it must add up to a *total* of 30 minutes or more per day and be done at least 5 days per week. For example, you could take one 30-minute walk or take three 10-minute walks for a daily total of 30 minutes.

	No	Yes
3. I currently engage in *regular* physical activity.	0	1
4. I have been *regularly* physically active for the past 6 months.	0	1

Note: You may want to cover the following scoring algorithm before reproducing this questionnaire for a client.

Scoring Algorithm

If (question 1 = 0 and question 2 = 0), then you are at stage 1.

If (question 1 = 0 and question 2 = 1), then you are at stage 2.

If (question 1 = 1 and question 3 = 0), then you are at stage 3.

If (question 1 = 1, question 3 = 1, and question 4 = 0), then you are at stage 4.

If (question 1 = 1, question 3 = 1, and question 4 = 1), then you are at stage 5.

From B. Marcus and L. Forsyth, 2009, *Motivating people to be physically active*, 2nd ed. (Champaign, IL: Human Kinetics). Reprinted, by permission, from B.H. Marcus et al., 1992, "The stages and processes of exercise adoption and maintenance in a worksite sample," *Health Psychology* 11: 386-395.

QUESTIONNAIRE 4.1 Processes of Change

Physical activity or exercise includes activities such as walking briskly, jogging, bicycling, swimming, and any other activity in which the exertion is at least as intense as these activities.

The following experiences can affect the exercise habits of some people. Think of any similar behaviors you may currently have or have had during the **past month.** Then rate how frequently the behavior occurs. Please circle the number that best describes your answer for each experience.

How frequently does this occur?

1 = never

2 = seldom

3 = occasionally

4 = often

5 = repeatedly

1. Instead of remaining inactive, I engage in some physical activity.   1 2 3 4 5

2. I tell myself I am able to be physically active if I want to.   1 2 3 4 5

3. I put things around my home to remind me to be physically active.   1 2 3 4 5

4. I tell myself that if I try hard enough, I can be physically active.   1 2 3 4 5

5. I recall information people have personally given me on the benefits of physical activity.   1 2 3 4 5

6. I make commitments to be physically active.   1 2 3 4 5

7. I reward myself when I am physically active.   1 2 3 4 5

8. I think about information from articles and advertisements on how to make physical activity a regular part of my life.   1 2 3 4 5

9. I keep things around my place of work that remind me to be physically active. 1 2 3 4 5

10. I find society changing in ways that make it easier to be physically active.   1 2 3 4 5

11. Warnings about the health hazards of inactivity affect me emotionally.   1 2 3 4 5

12. Dramatic portrayals of the evils of inactivity affect me emotionally.   1 2 3 4 5

13. I react emotionally to warnings about an inactive lifestyle.   1 2 3 4 5

14. I worry that inactivity can be harmful to my body.   1 2 3 4 5

15. I am considering the idea that regular physical activity would make me a healthier, happier person to be around.   1 2 3 4 5

16. I have someone I can depend on when I am having problems with physical activity.   1 2 3 4 5

17. I read articles about physical activity in an attempt to learn more about it.   1 2 3 4 5

18. I try to set realistic physical activity goals for myself rather than set myself up for failure by expecting too much.   1 2 3 4 5

(continued) ▶

19. I have a healthy friend who encourages me to be physically active when I don't feel up to it.   1 2 3 4 5

20. When I am physically active, I tell myself that I am being good to myself by taking care of my body.   1 2 3 4 5

21. The time I spend being physically active is my special time to relax and recover from the day's worries, not a task to get out of the way.   1 2 3 4 5

22. I am aware of more and more people encouraging me to be physically active these days.   1 2 3 4 5

23. I do something nice for myself for making efforts to be more physically active.   1 2 3 4 5

24. I have someone who points out my rationalizations for not being physically active.   1 2 3 4 5

25. I have someone who provides feedback about my physical activity.   1 2 3 4 5

26. I remove things that contribute to my inactivity.   1 2 3 4 5

27. I am the only one responsible for my health, and only I can decide whether or not I will be physically active.   1 2 3 4 5

28. I look for information related to physical activity.   1 2 3 4 5

29. I avoid spending long periods of time in environments that promote inactivity.   1 2 3 4 5

30. I feel that I would be a better role model for others if I were regularly physically active.   1 2 3 4 5

31. I think about the type of person I would be if I were physically active.   1 2 3 4 5

32. I notice that more businesses are encouraging their employees to be physically active by offering fitness courses and time off to work out.   1 2 3 4 5

33. I wonder how my inactivity affects those people who are close to me.   1 2 3 4 5

34. I realize that I might be able to influence others to be healthier if I would be more physically active.   1 2 3 4 5

35. I get frustrated with myself when I am not physically active.   1 2 3 4 5

36. I am aware that many health clubs now provide babysitting services to their members.   1 2 3 4 5

37. Some of my close friends might be more physically active if I were.   1 2 3 4 5

38. I consider the fact that I would feel more confident in myself if I were regularly physically active.   1 2 3 4 5

39. When I feel tired, I make myself be physically active anyway because I know I will feel better afterward.   1 2 3 4 5

40. When I'm feeling tense, I find physical activity a great way to relieve my worries.   1 2 3 4 5

From B. Marcus and L. Forsyth, 2009, *Motivating people to be physically active*, 2nd ed. (Champaign, IL: Human Kinetics). Reprinted, by permission, from B.H. Marcus et al., 1992, "The stages and processes of exercise adoption and maintenance in a worksite sample," *Health Psychology* 11: 386-395.

QUESTIONNAIRE 4.2 Confidence (Self-Efficacy)

Physical activity or exercise includes activities such as walking briskly, jogging, bicycling, swimming, and any other activity in which the exertion is at least as intense as these activities.

Circle the number that indicates how confident you are that you could be physically active in each of the following situations:

Scale

1 = not at all confident
2 = slightly confident
3 = moderately confident
4 = very confident
5 = extremely confident

1. When I am tired	1	2	3	4	5
2. When I am in a bad mood	1	2	3	4	5
3. When I feel I don't have time	1	2	3	4	5
4. When I am on vacation	1	2	3	4	5
5. When it is raining or snowing	1	2	3	4	5

From B. Marcus and L. Forsyth, 2009, *Motivating people to be physically active*, 2nd ed. (Champaign, IL: Human Kinetics). Reprinted with permission from *Research Quarterly for Exercise and Sport*, Vol. 63, pgs. 60-66. Copyright 1992 by the American Alliance for Health, Physical Education, Recreation and Dance, 1900 Association Drive, Reston, VA 20191.

QUESTIONNAIRE 4.3 Social Support for Physical Activity Scale

The following questions refer to social support for your physical activity.

The following is a list of things people might do or say to someone who is trying to do physical activity regularly. Please read and answer every question. If you are not physically active, then some of the questions may not apply to you.

Please rate each question *twice*. Under "Family," rate how often anyone living in your household has said or done what is described during the past 3 months. Under "Friends," rate how often your friends, acquaintances, or coworkers have said or done what is described during the past 3 months.

Please write *one* number from the following rating scale in each space:

    1 = none
    2 = rarely
    3 = a few times
    4 = often
    5 = very often
    0 = does not apply

	Family	Friends
1. Did physical activities with me		
2. Offered to do physical activities with me		
3. Gave me helpful reminders to be physically active (e.g., "Are you going to do your activity tonight?")		
4. Gave me encouragement to stick with my activity program		
5. Changed their schedule so we could do physical activities together		
6. Discussed physical activity with me		
7. Complained about the time I spend doing physical activity		
8. Criticized me or made fun of me for doing physical activities		
9. Gave me rewards for being physically active (e.g., gave me something I liked)		
10. Planned for physical activities on recreational outings		
11. Helped plan events around my physical activities		
12. Asked me for ideas on how they can be more physically active		
13. Talked about how much they like to do physical activity		

From B. Marcus and L. Forsyth, 2009, *Motivating people to be physically active*, 2nd ed. (Champaign, IL: Human Kinetics). Reprinted from *Preventive Medicine*, Vol. 16, J.F. Sallis et al., "The development of scales to measure social support for diet and exercise behaviors," pgs. 825-836. Copyright 1987, with permission from Elsevier.

QUESTIONNAIRE 4.4 Decisional Balance

Physical activity or exercise includes activities such as walking briskly, jogging, bicycling, swimming, and any other activity in which the exertion is at least as intense as these activities.

Please rate how important each of these statements is in your decision of whether to be physically active. In each case, think about how you feel **right now,** not how you have felt in the past or would like to feel.

Scale

1 = not at all important
2 = slightly important
3 = moderately important
4 = very important
5 = extremely important

1. I would have more energy for my family and friends
   if I were regularly physically active.   1 2 3 4 5

2. Regular physical activity would help me relieve tension.   1 2 3 4 5

3. I think I would be too tired to do my daily work after being physically active.   1 2 3 4 5

4. I would feel more confident if I were regularly physically active.   1 2 3 4 5

5. I would sleep more soundly if I were regularly physically active.   1 2 3 4 5

6. I would feel good about myself if I kept my commitment
   to be regularly physically active.   1 2 3 4 5

7. I would find it difficult to find a physical activity that I enjoy
   and that is not affected by bad weather.   1 2 3 4 5

8. I would like my body better if I were regularly physically active.   1 2 3 4 5

9. It would be easier for me to perform routine physical tasks
   if I were regularly physically active.   1 2 3 4 5

10. I would feel less stressed if I were regularly physically active.   1 2 3 4 5

11. I feel uncomfortable when I am physically active
    because I get out of breath and my heart beats very fast.   1 2 3 4 5

12. I would feel more comfortable with my body
    if I were regularly physically active.   1 2 3 4 5

13. Regular physical activity would take too much of my time.   1 2 3 4 5

14. Regular physical activity would help me have a more positive outlook on life.   1 2 3 4 5

15. I would have less time for my family and friends
    if I were regularly physically active.   1 2 3 4 5

16. At the end of the day, I am too exhausted to be physically active.   1 2 3 4 5

From B. Marcus and L. Forsyth, 2009, *Motivating people to be physically active*, 2nd ed. (Champaign, IL: Human Kinetics). Reprinted, by permission, from B.H. Marcus, W. Rakowski, and J.S. Rossi, 1992, "Assessing motivational readiness and decision-making for exercise," *Health Psychology* 11: 257-261.

QUESTIONNAIRE 4.5 Outcome Expectations for Exercise

The following are statements about the benefits of exercise (walking, jogging, swimming, biking, stretching, or lifting weights). Circle the number representing the degree to which you agree or disagree with these statements.

1. Makes me feel better physically   1 2 3 4 5

2. Makes my mood better in general   1 2 3 4 5

3. Helps me feel less tired   1 2 3 4 5

4. Makes my muscles stronger   1 2 3 4 5

5. Is an activity I enjoy doing   1 2 3 4 5

6. Gives me a sense of personal accomplishment   1 2 3 4 5

7. Makes me more alert mentally   1 2 3 4 5

8. Improves my endurance in performing my daily activities (such as
   personal care, cooking, shopping, light cleaning, taking out garbage) 1 2 3 4 5

9. Helps to strengthen my bones   1 2 3 4 5

From B. Marcus and L. Forsyth, 2009, *Motivating people to be physically active*, 2nd ed. (Champaign, IL: Human Kinetics). Reprinted, by permission, from B. Resnick et al., 2000, "Outcome expectations for exercise scale: Utility and psychometrics," *Journal of Gerontology: Social Sciences* 55B: S352-S356.

QUESTIONNAIRE 4.6 Physical Activity Enjoyment Scale

Please rate how you feel at the moment about physical activity. Below is a list of feelings with respect to physical activity. For each feeling, please mark the number that best describes you.

	1	2	3	4	5	6	7	
1. I enjoy it.								I hate it.
2. I feel bored.								I feel interested.
3. I dislike it.								I like it.
4. I find it pleasurable.								I find it unpleasurable.
5. I am very absorbed in physical activity.								I am not at all absorbed in physical activity.
6. It's no fun at all.								It's a lot of fun.
7. I find it energizing.								I find it tiring.
8. It makes me depressed.								It makes me happy.
9. It's very pleasant.								It's very unpleasant.
10. I feel good physically while doing it.								I feel bad physically while doing it.
11. It's very invigorating.								It's not at all invigorating.
12. I am very frustrated by it.								I am not at all frustrated by it.
13. It's very gratifying.								It's not at all gratifying.
14. It's very exhilarating.								It's not at all exhilarating.
15. It's not at all stimulating.								It's very stimulating.
16. It gives me a strong sense of accomplishment.								It does not give me any sense of accomplishment.
17. It's very refreshing.								It's not at all refreshing.
18. I would rather be doing something else.								There is nothing else I would rather be doing.

From B. Marcus and L. Forsyth, 2009, *Motivating people to be physically active*, 2nd ed. (Champaign, IL: Human Kinetics). Adapted, by permission, from D. Kendzierski and K.J. DeCarlo, 1991, "Physical activity enjoyment scale: Two validation studies," *Journal of Sport & Exercise Psychology* 13(1): 62-63.

QUESTIONNAIRE 7.1   Physical Activity History

If you do *not* currently participate in physical activity, answer these questions:

1. How long has it been since you did *regular* physical activity or exercise?
   a. Less than 6 months
   b. More than 6 months but less than 1 year
   c. More than 1 year but less than 2 years
   d. More than 2 years but less than 5 years
   e. More than 5 years but less than 10 years
   f. More than 10 years
   g. I have never been regularly physically active.

If you are *currently* physically active, answer the following questions:

1. How many days per week are you physically active? _____.
2. Approximately how many minutes are you physically active each time? _____.
3. How long have you been physically active at this level? _____.
4. What activities do you do? _____.

Answer the following questions whether or not you are currently physically active.

1. As an adult, were there ever times when you were physically active regularly for at least 3 months and then stopped being physically active for at least 3 months?
   a. Yes
   b. No
2. If yes, how many times? _____.
3. Regarding the most recent time, why did you stop your activity? (Please check as many as apply.)

Lack of time because of

___ Work or school	___ Lack of physical activity partner
___ Household duties	___ Lack of interest in physical activity
___ Children	___ Health problems
___ Social activities	___ Injury
___ Spouse	___ Season or weather change
___ Lack of money	___ Personal stress
___ Lack of facilities	Other: _____

From B. Marcus and L. Forsyth, 2009, *Motivating people to be physically active*, 2nd ed. (Champaign, IL: Human Kinetics).

APPENDIX B

The following is a list of organizations, suggested readings, and helpful Web sites you can use to enhance your programs.

Organizations

American College of Sports Medicine (ACSM)
www.acsm.org/sportsmed

American Heart Association National Center
www.americanheart.org

Centers for Behavioral and Preventive Medicine
E-mail: LSExercise@lifespan.org

Centers for Disease Control and Prevention (CDC)
www.cdc.gov/nccdphp/dnpa

The Cooper Institute
www.cooperinst.org

Stanford Health Promotion Resource Center (HPRC)
http://hprc.stanford.edu

Human Kinetics
www.HumanKinetics.com

National Heart, Lung, and Blood Institute (NHLBI)
www.nhlbi.nih.gov/

President's Council on Physical Fitness and Sports (PCPFS)
E-mail: cspain@osophs.dhhs.gov

Suggested Readings

A collection of physical activity questionnaires for health-related research. (1997). *Medicine and Science in Sports and Exercise, 29*(Suppl. 6).

American College of Sports Medicine. (1995). *Guidelines for exercise testing and prescription* (5th ed.). Baltimore: Williams & Wilkins.

Blair, S.N., Dunn, A.L., Marcus, B.H., Carpenter, R.A., & Jaret, P. (2001). *Active Living Every Day: 20 Weeks to Lifelong Vitality.* Champaign, IL: Human Kinetics.

Bouchard, C., Shephard, R., & Stephens, T. (1993). *Physical activity, fitness, and health: International proceedings and consensus statement.* Champaign, IL: Human Kinetics.

Centers for Disease Control. (1999). *Promoting physical activity: A guide for community action.* Champaign, IL: Human Kinetics.

Glaros, T.E. (1997). *Health promotion ideas that work: 84 proven activities for the workplace.* Champaign, IL: Human Kinetics.

Marcus, B.H., Owen, N., Forsyth, L.H., Cavill, N.A. & Fridinger, F. (1998). Physical activity interventions using mass media, print media, and information technology. *American Journal of Preventive Medicine 15*(4), 362-378.

Measurement of physical activity [Special issue]. (2000). *Research Quarterly for Exercise and Sport, 71.*

U.S. Department of Health and Human Services. (1996). *Physical activity and health: A report of the Surgeon General.* Atlanta, GA: Centers for Disease Control and Prevention, National Center for Chronic Disease Prevention and Health Promotion.

Web Sites

Choose to Move, American Heart Association: www.choosetomove. org

- *Information* (how to find target heart rate, how to exercise safely)
- *Assessment* (fitness level, BMI, target heart rate)
- *Strategies for change* (self-monitoring, goal setting)

Shape Up America: www.Shapeup.org

- *Information* (fitness glossary, physical activity IQ test)
- *Assessment* (fitness, strength, aerobic fitness)
- *Strategies for change* (benefits of physical activity, overcoming barriers)

Mayo Clinic Fitness and Sports Medicine Center: www.mayoclinic. com/health/fitness/SM99999

- *Information* (how to plan and start an exercise program, budgeting costs, strength training and stretching tips, injury prevention, sample walking programs)
- *Assessment* (fitness level, fitness awareness, BMI)
- *Strategies for change* (benefits of physical activity, overcoming barriers)

American Academy of Family Physicians: http://familydoctor.org/ healthfacts/059/

- *Information* (how to plan and start an exercise program, injury prevention, aerobic exercise, weight training)
- *Assessment* (target heart rate)
- *Strategies for change* (self-monitoring, social support, relapse prevention)

American Council on Exercise: http://www.acefitness.org/aboutace

- *Information* (safe and effective ways to exercise)
- *Strategies for change* (benefits of physical activity)

ACSM Health and Fitness Information: www.acsm.org/ health%2Bfitness/index.htm

- *Information* (active aging tips, guidelines for aerobic activity and getting started with exercise)
- *Assessment* (target heart rate)
- *Strategies for change* (social support)

REFERENCES

Chapter 1

American College of Sports Medicine. (2000). *ACSM's guidelines for exercise testing and prescription* (6th ed.). Philadelphia, PA: Lippincott Williams & Wilkins.

Barnes, P.M., & Schoenborn, C.A. (2003). *Physical activity among adults: United States, 2000.* Atlanta, GA: U.S. Department of Health and Human Services, Centers for Disease Control and Prevention, National Center for Health Statistics.

Caspersen, C.J. (1989). Physical activity epidemiology: Concepts, methods, and applications to exercise science. *Exercise and Sport Sciences Reviews, 17,* 423-473.

DeBusk, R.F., Stenestrand, U., Sheehan, M., & Haskell, W.L. (1990). Training effects of long versus short bouts of exercise in healthy subjects. *American Journal of Cardiology, 65,* 1010-1013.

Ebisu, T. (1985). Splitting the distance of endurance running on cardiovascular endurance and blood lipids. *Japanese Journal of Physical Education, 30,* 37-43.

Fletcher, G.F., Blair, S.N., Blumenthal, J., Caspersen, C., Chaitman, B., Epstein, S., et al. (1992). *American Heart Association position statement on exercise.* Dallas: American Heart Association.

Haskell, W.L., Lee, I.M., et al. (2007). Physical activity and public health. Updated recommendation for adults from the American College of Sports Medicine and the American Heart Association. *Medicine and Science in Sports and Exercise, 39,* 1423-1434.

King, A.C., Haskell, W.L., Taylor, C.B., Kraemer, H.C., & DeBusk, R.F. (1991). Group vs. home-based exercise training in healthy older men and women. *Journal of the American Medical Association, 266,* 1535-1542.

Marcus, B.H., Lewis, B.A., Williams, D.M., Dunsiger, S.I., Jakicic, J.M., Whiteley, J.A., Albrecht, A.E., Napolitano, M.A., Bock, B.C., Tate, D.F., Sciamanna, C.A., & Parisi, A.F. (2007a). A comparison of Internet and print-based physical activity interventions. *Archives of Internal Medicine, 167*(9), 944-949.

Marcus, B.H., Lewis, B.A., Williams, D.M., Whiteley, J. A., Albrecht, A.E., Jakicic, J.M., Parisi, A.F., Hogan, J.W., Napolitano, M.A., & Bock, B.C. (2007). Step into motion: A randomized trial examining the relative efficacy of Internet vs. print-based physical activity interventions. *Contemporary Clinical Trials,* 28(6):737-47.

Marcus, B.H., Napolitano, M.A., King, A.C., Lewis, B.A., Whiteley, J.A., Albrecht, A., Parisi, A., Bock, B., Pinto, B., Sciamanna, C., Jakicic, J., & Papandonatos, G. (2007). Telephone versus print delivery of an individualized motivationally tailored physical activity intervention: Project STRIDE. *Health Psychology, 26,* 401-409.

Marcus, B.H., Napolitano, M.A., Lewis, B.A., King, A.C., Whiteley, J.A., Albrecht, A.E., Parisi, A.F., Pinto, B.M., Bock, B.C., Sciamanna, C.A., Jakicic, J.M., & Papandonatos, G.D. (2007b). Examination of print and telephone channels for physical activity promotion: Rationale, design, and baseline data from project STRIDE. *Contemporary Clinical Trials, 28*(1), 90-104.

Marcus, B.H., Nigg, C.R., Riebe, D., & Forsyth, L.H. (2000). Interactive communication strategies: Implications for population-based physical activity promotion. *American Journal of Preventive Medicine, 19*(2), 121-126.

Marcus, B.H., Williams, D.M., Dubbert, P.M., Sallis, J.R., King, A.C., Yancey, A.K., Franklin, B.A., Buchner, D., Daniels, S., & Claytor, R. (2006). Physical activity intervention studies: What we know and what we need to know. *Circulation, 114*(24), 2739-2752.

Nelson, M.E., Rejeski, W.J., Blair, S.N., Duncan, P.W., Judge, J.O., King, A.C., Macera, C.A., & Castaneda-Sceppa, C. (2007). Physical activity and public health in older adults. Recommendation from the American College of Sports Medicine and the American Heart Association. *Circulation, 116*(9):1094-105.

NIH Consensus Development Panel on Physical Activity and Cardiovascular Health: NIH Consensus Conference. (1996). Physical activity and cardiovascular health. *Journal of the American Medical Association, 276,* 241-246.

Pate, R.R., Pratt, M., Blair, S.N., Haskell, W.L., Macera, C.A., Bouchard, C., et al. (1995). Physical activity and public health: A recommendation from the Centers for Disease Control and Prevention and the American College of Sports Medicine. *Journal of the American Medical Association, 273,* 402-407.

Prochaska, J.O., & DiClemente, C.C. (1983). The stages and processes of self-change in smoking: Towards an integrative model of change. *Journal of Consulting and Clinical Psychology, 51,* 390-395.

U.S. Department of Health and Human Services. (1996). *Physical activity and health: A report of the Surgeon General.* Atlanta, GA: Centers for Disease Control and Prevention, National Center for Chronic Disease Prevention and Health Promotion.

U.S. Department of Health and Human Services. (2000). *Healthy People 2010.* Washington, DC: U.S. Department of Health and Human Services. *Healthy People 2010.* 2nd ed. With Understanding and Improving Health and Objectives for Improving Health. 2 vols. Washington, DC: U.S. Government Printing Office, November 2000.

U.S. Department of Health and Human Services & U.S. Department of Agriculture. (2005). *Dietary guidelines for Americans, 2005* (6th ed.). Washington, DC: U.S. Government Printing Office.

Chapter 2

Bandura, A. (1986). *Social foundations of thought and action: A social cognitive theory.* Englewood Cliffs, NJ: Prentice Hall.

Bandura, A. (1977). Self-efficacy: Toward a unifying theory of behavior change. *Psychological Reviews, 84,* 192-215.

Bandura, A. (1997). *Self-efficacy: The exercise of control.* New York: H. Freeman.

Dunn, A.L., Marcus, B.H., Kampert, J.B., Garcia, M.E., Kohl, H.W., III, & Blair, S.N. (1997). Reduction in cardiovascular disease risk factors: 6-month results from Project Active. *Preventive Medicine, 26,* 883-892.

Haskell, W.L., Lee, I.M., et al. (2007). Physical activity and public health. Updated recommendation for adults from the American College of Sports Medicine and the American Heart Association. *Medicine and Science in Sports and Exercise, 39,* 1423-1434.

Janis, I.L., & Mann, L. (1977). *Decision making: A psychological analysis of conflict, choice and commitment.* New York: Free Press.

Marcus, B.H., Bock, B.C., Pinto, B.M., Forsyth, L.H., Roberts, M.B., & Traficante, R.M. (1998). Efficacy of an individualized, motivationally-tailored physical activity intervention. *Annals of Behavioral Medicine, 20,* 174-180.

Marcus, B.H., Rossi, J.S., Selby, V.C., Niaura, R.S., & Abrams, D.B. (1992). The stages and processes of exercise adoption and maintenance in a worksite sample. *Health Psychology, 11,* 386-395.

Marcus, B.H., Selby, V.C., Niaura, R.S., & Rossi, J.S. (1992).Self-efficacy and the stages of exercise behavior change. *Research Quarterly for Exercise and Sport, 63,* 60-66.

Marcus, B.H., & Simkin, L.R. (1993). The stages of exercise behavior. *Journal of Sports Medicine and Physical Fitness, 33,* 83-88.

Prochaska, J.O. (1979). *Systems of psychotherapy: A transtheoretical analysis.* Homewood, IL: Dorsey Press.

Prochaska, J.O., & DiClemente, C.C. (1983). The stages and processes of self-change in smoking: Towards an integrative model of change. *Journal of Consulting and Clinical Psychology, 51,* 390-395.

Prochaska, J.O., DiClemente, C.C., & Norcross, J.C. (1992). In search of how people change: Applications to addictive behaviors. *American Psychologist, 47,* 1102-1114.

Prochaska, J.O., Velicer, W.F., DiClemente, C.C., & Fava, J. (1988). Measuring processes of change: Applications to the cessation of smoking. *Journal of Consulting and Clinical Psychology, 56,* 520-528.

Skinner, B.F. (1953). *Science and human behavior.* New York: Free Press.

U.S. Department of Health and Human Services. (1996). *Physical activity and health: A report of the Surgeon General.* Atlanta, GA: Centers for Disease Control and Prevention, National Center for Chronic Disease Prevention and Health Promotion.

Chapter 3

Badland, H., & Schofield, G. (2005). Transport, urban design, and physical activity: An evidence-based update. *Transport Research Part D, 10,* 177-196.

Bandura, A. (1986). *Social foundations of thought and action: A social cognitive theory.* Englewood Cliffs, NJ: Prentice Hall.

Bandura, A. (1997). *Self-efficacy: The exercise of control.* New York: W.H. Freeman and Co.

Bandura, A. (2001). Social cognitive theory: An agentic perspective. *Annual Review of Psychology, 52,* 1-26.

Brownell, K.D., Stunkard, A.J., & Albaum, J.M. (1980). Evaluation and modification of exercise patterns in the natural environment. *American Journal of Psychiatry, 137,* 1540-1545.

Epstein, L.H. (1998). Integrating theoretical approaches to promote physical activity. *American Journal of Preventive Medicine, 15,* 257-265.

Glanz, K., & Rimer, B.K. (1995). *Theory at a glance: A guide for health promotion practice.* Bethesda, MD: U.S. Department of Health and Human Services, Public Health Service, National Institutes of Health, and National Cancer Institute.

Humpel, N., Owen, N., & Leslie, E. (2002). Environmental factors associated with adults' participation in physical activity. *American Journal of Preventive Medicine, 22*(3), 188-199.

Janis, I.L., & Mann, L. (1977). *Decision making: A psychological analysis of conflict, choice, and commitment.* New York: Collier Macmillan.

King, A.C., Blair, S.N., Bild, D.E., Dishman, R.K., Dubbert, P.M., Marcus, B.H., et al. (1992). Determinants of physical activity and interventions in adults. *Medicine and Science in Sports and Exercise, 24,* S221-S223.

Lewis, B.A., Marcus, B.H., Pate, R.P., & Dunn, A.L. (2002). Psychosocial mediators of physical activity behavior among adults and children. *American Journal of Preventive Medicine, 23*(2S), 26-35.

Marcus, B.H., Rakowski, W., & Rossi, J.S. (1992). Assessing motivational readiness and decision-making for exercise. *Health Psychology, 11,* 257-261.

Marcus, B.H., Selby, V.C., Niaura, R.S., & Rossi, J.S. (1992). Self-efficacy and the stages of exercise behavior change. *Research Quarterly for Exercise and Sport, 63,* 60-66.

Marlatt, G.A., & Gordon, J.R. (1985). *Relapse prevention: Maintenance strategies in the treatment of addictive behaviors.* New York: Guilford Press.

McLeroy, K.R., Bibeau, D., Steckler, A., & Glanz, K. (1988). An ecological perspective on health promotion programs. *Health Education Quarterly, 15,* 351-377.

Paffenbarger, R.S., Hyde, R.T., Wing, A.L., & Hsieh, C. (1986). Physical activity, all-cause mortality, and longevity of college alumni. *New England Journal of Medicine, 314,* 605-613.

Saelens, B.E., & Epstein, L.H. (1998). Behavioral engineering of activity choice in obese children. *International Journal of Obesity, 22,* 275-277.

Saelens, B.E., & Epstein, L.H. (1999). The rate of sedentary activities determines the reinforcing value of physical activity. *Health Psychology, 18,* 655-659.

Sallis, J.F., Bauman, A., & Pratt, M. (1998). Environmental and policy interventions to promote physical activity. *American Journal of Preventive Medicine, 15,* 379-397.

Sallis, J.F., Hovell, L.M.R., Hofstetter, C.R., Faucher, P., Elder, J.P., Blanchard, J., et al. (1989). A multivariate study of determinants of vigorous exercise in a community sample. *Preventive Medicine, 18*, 20-34.

Skinner, B.F. (1953). *Science and human behavior.* New York: Free Press.

U.S. Department of Health and Human Services. (1996). *Physical activity and health: A report of the Surgeon General.* Atlanta, GA: Centers for Disease Control and Prevention, National Center for Chronic Disease Prevention and Health Promotion.

Wankel, L.M. (1984). Decision-making and social support strategies for increasing exercise involvement. *Journal of Cardiac Rehabilitation, 4*, 124-135.

Chapter 4

Bandura, A. (1986). *Social foundations of thought and action: A social cognitive theory.* Englewood Cliffs, NJ: Prentice Hall.

Bandura, A. (1997). *Self-efficacy: The exercise of control.* New York: W.H. Freeman.

Baranowski, T., Anderson, C., & Carmack, C. (1998). Mediating variable framework in physical activity interventions: How are we doing? How might we do better? *American Journal of Preventive Medicine, 14*, 266-297.

Baron, R.M., & Kenny, D.A. (1986). The moderator–mediator variable distinction in social psychological research: Conceptual, strategic, and statistical considerations. *Journal of Personality and Social Psychology, 51*, 1173-1182.

Bauman, A.E., Sallis, J.F., Dzewaltowski, D.A., & Owen, N. (2002). Toward a better understanding of the influences on physical activity: The role of determinants, correlates, causal variables, mediators, moderators, and confounders. *American Journal of Preventive Medicine, 23*(2S), 5-14.

Blair, S.N., Dunn, A.L., Marcus, B.H., Carpenter, R.A., & Jaret, P. (2001). *Active living every day.* Champaign, IL: Human Kinetics.

Brassington, G.S., Atienza, A.A., Perczek, R.E., DiLorenzo, T.M., & King, A.C. (2002). Intervention-related cognitive versus social mediators of exercise adherence in the elderly. *American Journal of Preventive Medicine, 23*(2S), 80-86.

Cohen, S., Mermelstein, R., Kamarck, T., & Hoberman, H.M. (1985). Measuring the functional components of social support. In I.G. Sarason & B.R. Sarason (Eds.), *Social support: Theory, research, and applications* (pp. 73-94). The Hague: Martinus Nijhoff.

Courneya, K.S., & McAuley, E. (1995). Cognitive mediators of the social influence–exercise adherence relationship: A test of the theory of planned behavior. *Journal of Behavioral Medicine, 18,* 499-515.

DiClemente, C.C., Prochaska, J.O., Fairhurst, S.K., Velicer, W.F., Rossi, J.J., & Velasquez, M. (1991). The process of smoking cessation: An analysis of precontemplation, contemplation, and preparation stages of change. *Journal of Consulting and Clinical Psychology, 59*, 295-304.

Dishman, R.K., Motl, R.W., Saunders, R., Felton, G., Ward, D.S., Dowda, M., & Pate, R.R. (2005). Enjoyment mediates effects of a school-based physical activity intervention. *Medicine and Science in Sports and Exercise, 37*, 478-487.

Dunn, A.L., Marcus, B.H., Kampert, J.B., Garcia, M.E., Kohl, H.W., & Blair, S.N. (1997). Reduction in cardiovascular disease risk factors: 6-month results from Project Active. *Preventive Medicine, 26*, 883-892.

Hallam, J., & Petosa, R. (1998). A worksite intervention to enhance social cognitive theory constructs to promote exercise adherence. *American Journal of Health Promotion, 13*, 4-7.

Janis, I.L., & Mann, L. (1977). *Decision making: A psychological analysis of conflict, choice, and commitment.* New York: Collier Macmillan.

Kendzierski, D., & DeCarlo, K.J. (1991). Physical activity enjoyment scale: Two validation studies. *Journal of Sport and Exercise Psychology, 13*, 50-64.

King, A.C., Stokols, D., Talin, B., Brassington, G.S., & Killingsworth, R. (2002). Theoretical approaches to the promotion of physical activity: Forging a transdisciplinary paradigm. *American Journal of Preventive Medicine, 23*(2S), 15-25.

Leslie, E., Owen, N., Salmon, J., Bauman, A., Sallis, J.F., & Kai Lo, S. (1999). Insufficiently active Australian college students: Perceived personal, social, and environmental influences. *Preventive Medicine, 28,* 20-27.

Lewis, B.A., Marcus, B.H., Pate, R.R., & Dunn, A.L. (2002). Psychosocial mediators of physical activity behavior among adults and children. *American Journal of Preventive Medicine, 23,* 26-35.

Lewis, B.A., Forsyth, L.H., Pinto, B.M., Bock, B.C., Roberts, M., & Marcus, B.H. (2006). Psychosocial mediators of physical activity in a randomized controlled intervention trial. *Journal of Sport and Exercise Psychology, 28,* 193-204.

Marcus, B.H., Bock, B.C., Pinto, B.M., Forsyth, L.H., Roberts, M., & Traficante, R. (1998). Efficacy of individualized, motivationally tailored physical activity intervention. *Annals of Behavioral Medicine, 20,* 174-180.

Marcus, B.H., & Owen, N. (1992). Motivational readiness, self-efficacy and decision making for exercise. *Journal of Applied Social Psychology, 22*(1), 3-16.

Marcus, B.H., Rakowski, W., & Rossi, J.S. (1992). Assessing motivational readiness and decision-making for exercise. *Health Psychology, 11,* 257-261.

Marcus, B.H., Rossi, J.S., Selby, V.C., Niaura, R.S., & Abrams, D.B. (1992). The stages and processes of exercise adoption and maintenance in a worksite sample. *Health Psychology, 11,* 386-395.

Marcus, B.H., Selby, V.C., Niaura, R.S., & Rossi, J.S. (1992). Self-efficacy and the stages of exercise behavior change. *Research Quarterly for Exercise and Sport, 63,* 60-66.

Miller, Y.D., Trost, S.G., & Brown, W.J. (2002). Mediators of physical activity behavior change among women with young children. *American Journal of Preventive Medicine, 23*(2S), 98-103.

Miller, Y.D., Trost, S.G., & Brown, W.J. (2006). Will you take care of the kids? Mediating effects of partner support in changing physical activity among women with young children. *American Journal of Preventive Medicine, 23*(2S), 98-103.

Nichols, J.F., Willman, E., Caparosa, S., Sallis, J.F., Calfas, K.J., & Rowe, R. (2000). Impact of a worksite behavioral skills intervention. *American Journal of Health Promotion, 14,* 218-221.

Oka, R., King, A.C., & Young, D.R. (1995). Sources of social support as predictors of exercise adherence in women and men ages 50-65 years. *Women Health Research and Gender Policy, 1,* 161-175.

Pinto, B.M., Lynn, H., Marcus, B.H., DePue, J., & Goldstein, M.G. (2001). Physician-based activity counseling: Intervention effects on mediators of motivational readiness for exercise. *Annals of Behavioral Medicine, 23,* 2-10.

Prochaska, J.O., & DiClemente, C.C. (1983). Stages and processes of self-change of smoking: Toward an integrative model of change. *Journal of Consulting and Clinical Psychology, 51,* 390-395.

Resnick, B., Zimmerman, S.I., Orwig, D., Furstenberg, A., & Magaziner, J. (2000). Outcome expectations for exercise scale: Utility and psychometrics. *Journal of Gerontology: Social Sciences, 55B,* S352-S356.

Rosen, C.S. (2000). Is the sequencing of change processes by stage consistent across health problems? A meta-analysis. *Health Psychology, 19,* 593-604.

Rovniak, L.S., Anderson, E.S., Winett, R.A., & Stephens, R.S. (2002). Social cognitive determinants of physical activity in young adults: A prospective structural equation analysis. *Annals of Behavioral Medicine, 24,* 149-156.

Sallis, J.F., Calfas, K.J., Alcaraz, J.E., Gehrman, C., & Johnson, M.F. (1999). Potential mediators of change in a physical activity promotion course of university students: Project GRAD. *Annals of Behavioral Medicine, 21,* 149-158,

Sallis, J.F., Grossman, R.M., Pinski, R.B., Patterson, T.L., & Nader, P.R. (1987). The development of scales to measure social support for diet and exercise behaviors. *Preventive Medicine, 16,* 825-836.

Sallis, J.F., Pinski, R.B., Grossman, R.M., Patterson, T.L., & Nader, P.R. (1988). The development of self-efficacy scales for health-related diet and exercise behaviors. *Health Education Research, 3*(3), 283-292.

Sarason, I.G., & Sarason, B.R. (1985). *Social support: Theory, research, and applications.* The Hague: Martinus Nijhoff.

Steinhardt, M.A., & Dishman, R.K. (1989). Reliability and validity of expected outcomes and barriers for habitual physical activity. *Journal of Occupational Medicine, 31,* 536-546.

Stevens, M., Lemmink, K.A., de Greef, M.H., & Rispens, P. (2000). Gronigen Active Living Model (GALM): Stimulating physical activity in sedentary older adults; first results. *Preventive Medicine, 31,* 547-553.

Stoddard, A.M., Palombo, R., Troped, P.J., Sorensen, G. & Will, J.C. (2004). Cardiovascular disease risk reduction: The Massachusetts WISEWOMAN project. *Journal of Women's Health* (Larchmont), *13*(5), 539-546.

U.S. Department of Health and Human Services. (1996). *Physical activity and health: A report of the Surgeon General.* Atlanta, GA: Centers for Disease Control and Prevention, National Center for Chronic Disease Prevention and Health Promotion.

Wankel, L.M. (1993). The importance of enjoyment to adherence and psychological benefits from physical activity. *International Journal of Sport Psychology, 24,* 151-169.

Williams, D.M., Anderson, E.S., & Winett, R.A. (2005). A review of the outcome expectancy construct in physical activity research. *Annals of Behavioral Medicine, 29,* 70-79.

Williams, D.M., Papandonatos, G.D., Napolitano, M.A., & Lewis, B.A. (2006). Perceived enjoyment moderates the efficacy of an individually tailored physical activity intervention. *Journal of Sports and Exercise Psychology, 28,* 300-309.

Chapter 5

American Heart Association. (1984a). *Dancing for a healthy heart.* Dallas: Author.

American Heart Association. (1984b). *Running for a healthy heart.* Dallas: Author.

American Heart Association. (1984c). *Swimming for a healthy heart.* Dallas: Author.

American Heart Association. (1984d). *Walking for a healthy heart.* Dallas: Author.

American Heart Association. (1989). *Cycling for a healthy heart.* Dallas: Author.

Barnes, P.M., & Schoenborn, C.A. (2003). *Physical activity among adults: United States, 2000.* Advance data from vital and health statistics; no. 333. Hyattsville, MD: National Center for Health Statistics, 2003.

Bock, B.C., Marcus, B.H., Pinto, B., & Forsyth, L. (2001). Maintenance of physical activity following an individualized motivationally tailored intervention. *Annals of Behavioral Medicine, 23,* 79-87.

Dishman, R.K. (1994). *Advances in exercise adherence.* Champaign, IL: Human Kinetics.

Dunn, A.L., Garcia, M.E., Marcus, B.H., Kampert, J.B., Kohl, H.W., & Blair, S.N. (1998). Six-month physical activity and fitness changes in Project Active: A randomized trial. *Medicine and Science in Sports and Exercise, 30,* 1076-1083.

Dunn, A.L., Marcus, B.H., Kampert, J.B., Garcia, M.E., Kohl, H.W., III, & Blair, S.N. (1999). Comparison of lifestyle and structured interventions to increase physical activity and cardio-respiratory fitness: A randomized trial. *Journal of the American Medical Association, 281,* 327-334.

Fletcher, G.F., Blair, S.N., Blumenthal, J., Casperson, C., Chaitman, B., Epstein, S., et al. (1992). *American Heart Association position statement on exercise.* Dallas: American Heart Association.

Haskell, W.L., Lee, I.M., et al. (2007). Physical activity and public health. Updated recommendation for adults from the American College of Sports Medicine and the American Heart Association. *Medicine and Science in Sports and Exercise, 39,* 1423-1434.

Madden M. (2006). Reports: Internet evolution: Internet penetration and impact. PEW Internet and American Life Project. Retrieved August 9, 2006, from www.pewinternet.org/PPF/r/182/report_display.asp.

Marcus, B.H., Banspach, S.W., Lefebvre, R.C., Rossi, J.S., Carleton, R.A., & Abrams, D.B. (1992). Using the stages of change model to increase the adoption of physical activity among community participants. *American Journal of Health Promotion, 6,* 424-429.

Marcus, B.H., Bock, B.C., Pinto, B.M., Forsyth, L.H., Roberts, M.B., & Traficante, R.M. (1998). Efficacy of an individualized, motivationally-tailored physical activity intervention. *Annals of Behavioral Medicine, 20,* 174-180.

Marcus, B.H., Dubbert, P.M., Forsyth, L.H., McKenzie, T.L., Stone, E.J., Dunn, A.L., & Blair, S.N. (2000). Physical activity behavior change: Issues in adoption and maintenance. *Health Psychology, 19*(1), 32-41.

Marcus, B.H., Emmons, K.M., Simkin-Silverman, L.R., Linnan, L.A., Taylor, E.R., Bock, B.C., et al. (1998). Evaluation of motivationally tailored vs. standard self-help physical activity interventions at the workplace. *American Journal of Health Promotion, 12*, 246-253.

Marcus, B.H., Lewis, B.A., Williams, D.M., Dunsiger, S.I., Jakicic, J.M., Whiteley J.A., Albrecht, A.E., Napolitano, M.A., Bock, B.C., Tate, D.F., Sciamanna, C.A., & Parisi, A.F. (2007a). A comparison of Internet and print-based physical activity interventions. *Archives of Internal Medicine, 167*(9), 944-949.

Marcus, B.H., Lewis, B.A., Williams, D.M., Whiteley, J. A., Albrecht, A.E., Jakicic, J.M., Parisi, A.F., Hogan, J.W., Napolitano, M.A., & Bock, B.C. (2007b). Step Into Motion: A randomized trial examining the relative efficacy of Internet vs. print-based physical activity interventions. *Contemporary Clinical Trials, 28*(6), 737-747.

Marcus, B.H., Napolitano, M.A., King, A.C., Lewis, B.A., Whiteley, J.A., Albrecht, A.E., Parisi, A.F., Bock, B.C., Pinto, B.M., Sciamanna, C., Jakicic, J.M., & Papandonatos, G.D. (2007). Telephone versus print delivery of an individualized motivationally-tailored physical activity intervention: Project STRIDE. *Health Psychology, 26*(4), 401-409.

Marcus, B.H., Napolitano, M.A., Lewis, B.A., King, A.C., Whiteley, J.A., Albrecht, A.E., Parisi, A.F., Pinto, B.M., Bock, B.C., Sciamanna, C.A., Jakicic, J.M., & Papandonatos, G.D. (2007). Examination of print and telephone channels for physical activity promotion: Rationale, design, and baseline data from project STRIDE. *Contemporary Clinical Trials, 28*(1), 90-104.

Pate, R.R., Pratt, M., Blair, S.N., Haskell, W.L., Macera, C.A., Bouchard, C., et al. (1995). Physical activity and public health: A recommendation from the Centers for Disease Control and Prevention and the American College of Sports Medicine. *Journal of the American Medical Association, 273*, 402-407.

U.S. Department of Health and Human Services. *Healthy People 2010*. 2nd ed. With Understanding and Improving Health and Objectives for Improving Health. 2 vols. Washington, DC: U.S. Government Printing Office, November 2000.

U.S. Department of Health and Human Services. (1996). *Physical activity and health: A report of the Surgeon General*. Atlanta, GA: Centers for Disease Control and Prevention, National Center for Chronic Disease Prevention and Health Promotion.

Chapter 6

A collection of physical activity questionnaires for health-related research. (1997). *Medicine and Science in Sports and Exercise, 29*(Suppl. 6).

Borg, G. (1998). *Perceived exertion and pain scales*. Champaign, IL: Human Kinetics.

Haskell, W.L., Lee, I., Pate, R.R., Powell, K.E., Blair, S.N., Franklin, B.A., Macera, C.A., Heath, G.W., Thompson, P.D., & Bauman, A. (2007). Physical activity and public health: Updated recommendation for adults from the American College of Sports Medicine and the American Heart Association. *Medicine and Science in Sports and Exercise* [Special report], 1423-1434.

Heyward, V.H. (2006). *Advanced fitness assessment and exercise prescription* (5th ed.). Champaign, IL: Human Kinetics.

Marcus, B.H., & Simkin, L.R. (1993). The stages of exercise behavior. *Journal of Sports Medicine and Physical Fitness, 33*, 83-88.

Measurement of physical activity [Special issue]. (2000). *Research Quarterly for Exercise and Sport, 71*.

Welk, G.J., Differding, J.A., Thompson, R.W., Blair, S.N., Dziura, J., & Hart, P. (2000). The utility of the Digi-Walker step counter to assess daily physical activity patterns. *Medicine and Science in Sports and Exercise 32*(9), S481-S488.

Chapter 7

Blair, S.N., Dunn, A.L., Marcus, B.H., Carpenter, R.A., & Jaret, P. (2001). *Active living every day.* Champaign, IL: Human Kinetics.

Physical Activity Readiness Questionnaire (PAR-Q) © 2002. Canadian Society for Exercise Physiology. http://www.csep.ca.

Chapter 8

Bandura, A. (1986). *Social foundations of thought and action: A social cognitive theory.* Englewood Cliffs, NJ: Prentice Hall.

Bandura, A. (1997). *Self-efficacy: The exercise of control.* New York: W.H. Freeman and Co.

Blair, S.N., Dunn, A.L., Marcus, B.H., Carpenter, R.A., & Jaret, P. (2001). *Active living every day.* Champaign, IL: Human Kinetics.

Dunn, A.L., Garcia, M.E., Marcus, B.H., Kampert, J.B., Kohl, H.W., & Blair, S.N. (1998). Six-month physical activity and fitness changes in Project Active, a randomized trial. *Medicine and Science in Sports and Exercise, 30,* 1076-1083.

Dunn, A.L., Marcus, B.H., Kampert, J.B., Garcia, M.E., Kohl, H.W., III, & Blair, S.N. (1997). Reduction in cardiovascular disease risk factors: 6-month results from Project Active. *Preventive Medicine, 26,* 883-892.

Dunn, A.L., Marcus, B.H., Kampert, J.B., Garcia, M.E., Kohl, H.W., III, & Blair, S.N. (1999). Project Active: A 24-month randomized trial to compare lifestyle and structured physical activity interventions. *Journal of the American Medical Association, 281,* 327-334.

Haskell, W. L., Lee, I.M., et al. (2007). Physical activity and public health. Updated recommendation for adults from the American College of Sports Medicine and the American Heart Association. *Medicine and Science in Sports and Exercise, 39,* 1423-1434.

Marcus, B.H., Banspach, S.W., Lefebvre, R.C., Rossi, J.S., Carleton, R.A., & Abrams D.B. (1992). Using the stages of change model to increase the adoption of physical activity among community participants. *American Journal of Health Promotion, 6,* 424-429.

Marcus, B.H., Bock, B.C., Pinto, B.M., Forsyth, L.H., Roberts, M., & Traficante, R. (1998). Efficacy of individualized, motivationally tailored physical activity intervention. *Annals of Behavioral Medicine, 20,* 174-180.

Marcus, B.H., Emmons, K.M., Simkin-Silverman, L.R., Linnan, L.A., Taylor, E.R., Bock, B.C., et al. (1998). Evaluation of stage-matched versus standard self-help physical activity interventions at the workplace. *American Journal of Health Promotion, 12,* 246-253.

Marcus, B.H., Lewis, B.A., Williams, D.M., Dunsiger, S.I., Jakicic, J.M., Whiteley J.A., Albrecht A.E., Napolitano M.A., Bock, B.C., Tate, D.F., Sciamanna C.A., & Parisi, A.F. (2007). A comparison of Internet and print-based physical activity interventions. *Archives of Internal Medicine, 167*(9), 944-949.

Marcus, B.H., Napolitano, M.A., King, A.C., Lewis, B.A., Whiteley, J.A., Albrecht, A.E., Parisi, A.F., Bock, B.C., Pinto, B.M., Sciamanna, C., Jakicic, J.M., & Papandonatos, G.D. (2007). Telephone versus print delivery of an individualized motivationally-tailored physical activity intervention: Project STRIDE. *Health Psychology, 26*(4), 401-409.

Pate, R.R., Pratt, M., Blair, S.N., Haskell, W.L., Macera, C.A., Bouchard, C., et al. (1995). Physical activity and public health: A recommendation from the Centers for Disease Control and Prevention and the American College of Sports Medicine. *Journal of the American Medical Association, 273,* 402-407.

Prochaska, J.O., & DiClemente, C.C. (1983). The stages and processes of self-change in smoking: Towards an integrative model of change. *Journal of Consulting and Clinical Psychology, 51,* 390-395.

Rinne, M., & Toropainen, E. (1998). How to lead a group: Practical principles and experiences of conducting a promotional group in health-related physical activity. *Patient Education and Counseling, 33,* S69-S76.

U.S. Department of Health and Human Services. (1996). *Physical activity and health: A report of the Surgeon General.* Atlanta, GA: Centers for Disease Control and Prevention, National Center for Chronic Disease Prevention and Health Promotion.

Chapter 9

Chan, C.B., Ryan, D.A., & Tudor-Locke, C. (2004). Health benefits of a pedometer-based physical activity intervention in sedentary workers. *Preventive Medicine, 39,* 1215-1222.

Dishman, R.K., Oldenburg, B., O'Neal, H., & Shephard, R.J. (1998). Worksite physical activity interventions. *American Journal of Preventive Medicine, 15,* 344-361.

Glaros, T.E. (1997). *Health promotion ideas that work: 84 proven activities for the workplace.* Champaign, IL: Human Kinetics.

Marcus, B.H., Emmons, K.M., Simkin-Silverman, L.R., Linnan, L.A., Taylor, E.R., Bock, B.C., et al. (1998). Evaluation of stage-matched versus standard self-help physical activity interventions at the workplace. *American Journal of Health Promotion, 12,* 246-253.

Marshall, A.L., Owen, N., & Bauman, A.E. (2004). Mediated approaches for influencing physical activity: Update of the evidence on mass media, print, telephone and website delivery of interventions. *Journal of Science in Medicine and Sport, 7*(Suppl.), 74-80.

Proper, K.I., Hildebrandt, V.H., Van der Beek, A.J., Twisk, J.W., & Van Mechelen, W. (2003). Effect of individual counseling on physical activity fitness and health: A randomized controlled trial in a workplace setting. *American Journal of Preventive Medicine, 24,* 218-226.

Sharratt, M.T., & Cox, M. (1988). Employee fitness: State of the art. *Canadian Journal of Public Health, 79,*S40-S43.

Shephard, R.J. (1992). A critical analysis of work-site fitness programs and their postulated economic benefits. *Medicine and Science in Sports and Exercise,24,* 354-370.

U.S. Department of Health and Human Services. (1993). *1992 national survey of worksite health promotion activities.* Washington, DC: U.S. Government Printing Office.

U.S. Department of Health and Human Services, Public Health Service, Centers for Disease Control and Prevention, National Center for Chronic Disease Prevention and Health Promotion, & Division of Nutrition and Physical Activity. (1999). *Promoting physical activity: A guide for community action.* Champaign, IL: Human Kinetics.

Wanzel, R.S. (1994). Decades of worksite fitness programmes: Progress or rhetoric? *Sports Medicine, 17,* 324-337.

Chapter 10

Abrams, D.B. (1991). Conceptual models to integrate individual and public health interventions: The example of the workplace. In *Proceedings of the International Conference on Promoting Dietary Change in Communities* (pp. 170-190). Seattle: Fred Hutchinson Cancer Research Center.

Calfas, K.J., Sallis, J.F., Zabinski, M.F., et al. (2002). Preliminary evaluation of a multi-component program for nutrition and physical activity change in primary care: PACE+ for adults. *Preventive Medicine 34*(2), 153-161.

Cardinal, B.J., & Sachs, M.L. (1996). Effects of mail-mediated, stage-matched exercise behavior change strategies on female adults' leisure-time exercise behavior. *Journal of Sports Medicine and Physical Fitness, 36,* 100-107.

Dishman, R.K., & Buckworth, J. (1996). Increasing physical activity: A quantitative synthesis. *Medicine and Science in Sports and Exercise, 28,* 706-719.

Fox, S. (2006): Most internet users start at a search engine when looking for health information online. Very few check the source and date of the information they find. The PEW Internet & American Life Project. Available at www.pewinternet.org. October 29, 2006.

Heath, G.W., Brownson, R.C., Kruger, J., Miles, R., Powell, K.E., Ramsey, C.T., & the Task Force on Community Preventive Services (2006). The effectiveness of urban design and land use and transport policies and practices to increase physical activity: A systematic review. *Journal of Physical Activity and Health, 3*(Suppl. 1), S55-S76t.

Humpel, N., Owen, N., & Leslie, E. (2002). Environmental factors associated with adults' participation in physical activity: A review. *American Journal of Preventive Medicine, 22,* 188-199.

Jacobs, A.D., Ammerman, A.S., Ennett, S.T., Campbell, M.K., Tawney, K.W., Aytur, S.A., Marshall, S.W., Will, J.C., & Rosamond, W.D. (2004). Effects of a tailored follow-up intervention on health behaviors, beliefs, and attitudes. *Journal of Women's Health* (Larchmont), *13*(5), 557-568.

Kahn, E.B., Ramsey, L.T., Brownson, R.C., Heath, G.W., Howze, E.H., Powell, K.E., Stone, E.J., Rajab, M.W., & Corso, P. (2002). The effectiveness of interventions to increase physical activity: A systematic review. *American Journal of Preventive Medicine, 22,* 73-107.

King, A.C. (1998). How to promote physical activity in the community: Research experiences from the U.S. highlighting different community approaches. *Patient Education and Counseling, 33,* S3-S12.

King, A.C., Friedman, R., Marcus, B.H., Castro, C., Forsyth, L.H., Napolitano, M., et al. (2002). Harnessing motivational forces in the promotion of physical activity: The Community Health Advice by Telephone (CHAT) project. *Health Education Research* [Special issue], *17*(5), 627-636.

King, A.C., Friedman, R.H., Marcus, B.H., Castro, C., Napolitano, M., Ahn, D., & Baker, L. (2007). Ongoing physical activity advice by humans versus computers: The Community Health Advice by Telephone (CHAT) trial. *Health Psychology, 26*(6):718-727.

King, A.C., Haskell, W.L., Taylor, C.B., Kraemer, H.C., & DeBusk, R.F. (1991). Group vs. home-based exercise training in healthy older men and women. *Journal of the American Medical Association, 266,* 1535-1542.

King, A.C., Taylor, C.B., Haskell, W.L., & DeBusk, R.F. (1988). Strategies for increasing early adherence to and long-term maintenance of home-based exercise training in healthy middle-aged men and women. *American Journal of Cardiology, 61,* 628-632.

Kotler, P., & Zaltman, G. (1971). Social marketing: An approach to planned social change. *Journal of Marketing, 35,* 3-12.

Luepker, R.V., Murray, D.M., Jacobs, D.R., Jr., & Mittelmark, M.B. (1994). Community education for cardiovascular disease prevention: Risk factor changes in the Minnesota Heart Health Program. *American Journal of Public Health, 84,* 1383-1393.

Madden, M. (2006). Reports: Internet evolution. Internet penetration and impact. Pew Internet and American Life Project. Retrieved May 9, 2007, from www.pewinternet.org/PPF/r/182/report_display.asp.

Madden M, & Rainie, L. (2003): America's online pursuits: The changing picture of who's online and what they do. The Pew Internet & American Life Project. Available at www.pewinternet.org. December 28, 2003.

Marcus, B.H., Banspach, S.W., Lefebvre, R.C., Rossi, J.S., Carleton, R.A., & Abrams, D.B. (1992). Using the stages of change model to increase the adoption of physical activity among community participants. *American Journal of Health Promotion, 6,* 424-429.

Marcus, B.H., Bock, B.C., Pinto, B.M., Forsyth, L.H., Roberts, M., & Traficante, R. (1998). Efficacy of individualized, motivationally tailored physical activity intervention. *Annals of Behavioral Medicine, 20,* 174-180.

Marcus, B.H., Emmons, K.M., Simkin-Silverman, L.R., Linnan, L.A., Taylor, E.R., Bock, B.C., et al. (1998). Evaluation of stage-matched versus standard self-help physical activity interventions at the workplace. *American Journal of Health Promotion, 12,* 246-253.

Marcus, B.H., Lewis, B.A., Williams, D.M., Dunsiger, S I., Jakicic, J.M., Whiteley J.A., Albrecht, A.E., Napolitano, M.A., Bock, B.C., Tate, D.F., Sciamanna, CA., & Parisi, A.F. (2007). A comparison of Internet and print-based physical activity interventions. *Archives of Internal Medicine, 167*(9), 944-949.

Marcus, B.H., Napolitano, M.A., King, A.C., Lewis, B.A., Whiteley, J.A., Albrecht, A.E., Parisi, A.F., Bock, B.C., Pinto, B.M., Sciamanna, C., Jakicic, J.M., & Papandonatos, G.D. (2007). Telephone versus print delivery of an individualized motivationally-tailored physical activity intervention: Project STRIDE. *Health Psychology, 26*(4), 401-409.

Marcus, B.H., Nigg, C.R., Riebe, D., & Forsyth, L.H. (2000). Interactive, preventive communication strategies: A proactive approach for reaching out to large populations. *American Journal of Health Promotion, 19*(2), 121-126.

Marcus, B.H., Owen, N., Forsyth, L.H., Cavill, N.A., & Fridinger, F. (1998). Physical activity interventions using mass media, print media, and information technology. *American Journal of Preventive Medicine, 15,* 362-378.

Marshall, A.L., Owen, N., & Bauman, A.E. (2004). Mediated approaches for influencing physical activity: Update of the evidence on mass media, print, telephone and website delivery of interventions. *Journal of Science, Medicine, & Sport, 7*(Suppl.), 74-80.

McLeroy, K.R., Bibeau, D., Steckler, A., & Glanz, K. (1998). An ecological perspective on health promotion programs. *Health Education Quarterly, 15,* 351-377.

Pinto, B.M., Friedman, R., Marcus, B., Ling, T., Tennstedt, S., and Gillman, M. (2000) Physical activity promotion using a computer-based telephone counseling system. *Annals of Behavioral Medicine, 22,* S212 (abstr.).

Rees, T. (2005). More Americans going online looking for health information. *Profiles in Healthcare Marketing, 21*(4), 2.

Staten, L.K., Gregory-Mercado, K.Y., Ranger-Moore, J., Will, J.C., Giuliano, A.R., Ford, E.S., & Marshall, J. (2004). Provider counseling, health education, and community health workers: The Arizona WISEWOMAN project. *Journal of Women's Health* (Larchmont), *13*(5), 547-556.

Stoddard, A.M., Palombo, R., Troped, P.J., Sorensen, G., & Will, J.C. (2004). Cardiovascular disease risk reduction: The Massachusetts WISEWOMAN project. *Journal of Women's Health* (Larchmont), *13*(5), 539-546.

U.S. Department of Health and Human Services, Public Health Service, Centers for Disease Control and Prevention, National Center for Chronic Disease Prevention and Health Promotion, & Division of Nutrition and Physical Activity. (1999). *Promoting physical activity: A guide for community action.* Champaign, IL: Human Kinetics.

Will, J.C., Farris, R.P., Sander, C.G., Stockmyer, C.K., & Finklestein, E.A. (2004). Health promotion interventions for disadvantaged women: Overview of the WISEWOMAN projects. *Journal of Women's Health* (Larchmont), *13*(5), 484-502.

Young, D.R., Haskell, W.L., Taylor, C.B., & Fortmann, S.P. (1996). Effect of community health education on physical activity knowledge, attitudes, and behavior. *American Journal of Epidemiology, 144,* 264-274.

INDEX

ABOUT THE AUTHORS

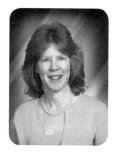

Bess H. Marcus, PhD, is a professor in the departments of community health and psychiatry and human behavior at the Alpert Medical School of Brown University and director of the Centers for Behavioral and Preventive Medicine at the Miriam Hospital. Dr. Marcus is a clinical health psychologist who has spent the past 20 years conducting research on physical activity behavior and has published more than 150 papers and book chapters as well as three books on this topic.

Dr. Marcus has developed a series of assessment instruments to measure psychosocial mediators of physical activity behavior and has also developed low-cost interventions to promote physical activity behavior in community, workplace, and primary care settings. Dr. Marcus has participated in panels for the American Heart Association, American College of Sports Medicine, Centers for Disease Control and Prevention, and National Institutes of Health; these panels have created recommendations regarding the quantity and intensity of physical activity necessary for health benefits. Marcus was also a contributing author to the *Surgeon General's Report on Physical Activity and Health*. She served as an advisor on the curriculum development for Project Active and is a coauthor of *Active Living Every Day* (Human Kinetics). Marcus is recognized internationally for her outstanding research in helping people to become more physically active and has spoken on this topic worldwide.

Marcus makes time to be physically active on most days of the week. She enjoys walking, swimming, and cycling with her husband, Dan, her three children, and friends.

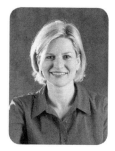

LeighAnn Forsyth, PhD, is a clinical health psychologist. She has a private practice specializing in weight management, body image, and women's health. She also is an adjunct professor of psychology at Cleveland State University, where she conducts research on physical activity adoption and lectures on behavior modification.

During a clinical internship and two-year postdoctoral fellowship at the Brown University Center for Behavioral and Preventive Medicine at the Miriam Hospital, Forsyth participated in several research programs applying the stages of motivational readiness to promote physical activity adoption.

She has published several professional articles and book chapters on physical activity promotion and the stages of motivational readiness and serves as a consultant on physical activity research grants. Forsyth is a member of the Society of Behavioral Medicine and the Association for the Advancement of Behavior Society.

With three young children, Forsyth receives a daily dose of physically active parenting. She also enjoys jogging, hiking, playing tennis, and biking. She and her husband, Paul, and their children reside in Shaker Heights, Ohio.